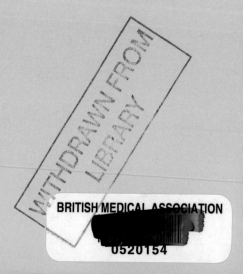

Hair Care

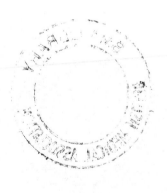

Hair Care
An Illustrated Dermatologic Handbook

Zoe Diana Draelos MD
Clinical Associate Professor
Department of Dermatology
Wake Forest University School of Medicine
Winston-Salem, NC, USA

and

Dermatology Consulting Services
High Point, NC, USA

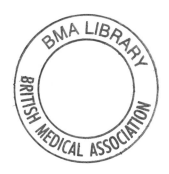

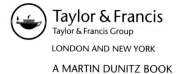

Taylor & Francis
Taylor & Francis Group

LONDON AND NEW YORK

A MARTIN DUNITZ BOOK

© 2005 Taylor & Francis, an imprint of Taylor & Francis Group

First published in the United Kingdom in 2005
by Taylor & Francis, an imprint of the Taylor & Francis Group, 2 Park Square, Milton Park, Abingdon, Oxon OX14 4RN

Tel.:   +44 (0) 20 7017 6000
Fax.:   +44 (0) 20 7017 6699
E-mail: info@dunitz.co.uk
Website: http://www.dunitz.co.uk

A CIP record for this book is available from the British Library.

Library of Congress Cataloguing-in-Publication Data

Data available on application

ISBN 1 84184 194 3

Distributed in North and South America by

Taylor & Francis
2000 NW Corporate Blvd
Boca Raton, FL 33431, USA

Within Continental USA
Tel: 800 272 7737;   Fax: 800 374 3401
Outside Continental USA
Tel: 561 994 0555;   Fax: 561 361 6018
E-mail: orders@crcpress.com

Distributed in the rest of the world by
Thomson Publishing Services
Cheriton House
North Way
Andover, Hampshire SP10 5BE, UK
Tel.:   +44 (0)1264 332424
E-mail: salesorder.tandf@thomsonpublishingservices.co.uk

Composition by J&L Composition, Filey, North Yorkshire

Printed and bound in Italy by Printer Trento

DEDICATION

To my two boys, Mark and Matthew, whose hair I have cut since birth.

Foreword

Patients expect their dermatologists to be knowledgeable in all issues related to the science of hair care. However, none of this information is routinely taught in dermatology programs. As a result there has always been a huge void for a textbook on hair care as it relates to clinical practice. Dr Zoe Draelos's book, *Hair Care: An Illustrated Dermatologic Handbook*, finally fills this void.

Zoe Diana Draelos is a committed clinician/scientist who has dedicated her professional career researching cosmetics in dermatology. She is one of the most respected authorities on the subject. Dermatologists around the globe seek her advice on what is the best for their patients from an efficacy as well as a safety point of view. Industry routinely consults her for her views on optimal and safe dermatological formulations. She is one of the most sought after speakers on the topic not only because of her great knowledge but also because of her clarity and enthusiasm. She is a former Rhodes Scholar and has become one of the most prolific dermatologists in the world.

Dr Draelos has now authored one of the most comprehensive textbooks devoted to hair cosmetics. This is the first book solely written by a dermatologist on the science of hair care. It bridges the gap between hair cosmetic basic science, salon practice hair care and finally what the practicing dermatologist sees in his/her practice. The linking of these three areas is crucial for the optimal beautification of the patient's hair. Dr Draelos's combined medical and engineering background gives her a unique and in-depth insight into the mechanics of hair breakage, noninvasive testing of hair fragility, and physico-chemical properties of hair. She has taken this information, simplified it, and made it absolutely crystal clear for the practitioner. Her writing style flows wonderfully and makes this text easy to read for anyone interested in the science of hair care. The information in the book is most practical and will allow the clinician to answer some of the most difficult questions patients ask. The book is rich in photographs that further add to our understanding of hair and what our patients do to it. Grooming, coloring, straightening, and curling are all covered in great detail in an organized lucid manner. The reason why shampoos and conditioners contain certain components is logically explained. The whole spectrum of hair loss and hair growth as it relates to cosmetic science is covered. In short, this book is a treasure and will be referred to for many years to come.

Jerry Shapiro MD FRCPC
Clinical Professor
Division of Dermatology
University of British Columbia
Vancouver, British Columbia
Canada

Acknowledgments

This text would not have been possible without the contributions of time and talent from many individuals. I would like to thank the hair research laboratory at Procter & Gamble for the numerous electron micrographs that are displayed in this text. Their state-of-the-art facilities produced these images, which were borrowed to help the reader see aspects of hair far beyond the reaches of the human eye. I am also indebted to David Bernens, Manager of External Relations, Procter & Gamble, who has provided inspiration and technical assistance to facilitate the gathering of much of the knowledge present in this text, which is only available in corporate archives. Other individuals at Procter & Gamble who spent their valuable time educating me include Lauren Thaman-Hodges, Sherrie McMaster, Dianna Kenneally, and Jim Monton.

I am indebted to my good friends Peggie and Roger Powell, and Michael and Phillip of Chisara's salon in High Point, North Carolina, who helped with much of the salon photography presented in the text. I also want to say a special thank you to Marcia Smith and Marissa who let me into their own home to obtain pictures. These individuals provided the extra hands, models, and ideas to make the art of hair care come to life as part of an educational story.

I would also like to thank my husband Michael and my son Mark who helped with the digital image processing necessary to create many of the images presented here. Lastly, I would like to thank my son Matthew who helped me organize, file, print, and punch during the development of the text. An illustrated book is a compilation of knowledge, images, computer graphics, and words. None of this could have been accomplished without the help of many who believed that this project deserved merit.

Contents

Introduction

Hair. It defines who we are in our eyes and shapes others' perceptions of us. We are classified as bald or bushy or thinning or luxuriant when it comes to our hair. Hair sits predominantly on top of our heads providing little but cosmetic adornment, yet poems, songs, and stories are written about hair. Children learn about the folk story of Rapunzel who let down her long golden hair for her suitor to climb into her tower of imprisonment. We sing about Sampson in the Old Testament of the Bible who lost his strength when he was tricked into allowing Delilah to cut his hair. We remember the O'Henry story *The Gift of the Magi* where the wife cut her lovely long hair to purchase a pocket watch chain for her husband, while the husband sold his pocket watch to purchase some beautiful combs for his wife's long hair. We marvel at the irony of the woman who loved her husband so much that she cut her precious hair.

Hair seems to be a fascination. We cut it, style it, curl it, straighten it, lighten it, darken it, comb it, wash it, dry it, and cry about it. Hair is the topic of this book – a long time academic interest of mine. I have had several varied opportunities to think about hair through the years. While in high school, I had the opportunity to look at hair through the eyes of a cosmetologist, learning to cut clumps of hair shafts into the fashion of the moment. It is this expertise that I draw upon when discussing the cosmetic aspects of hair alterations. During my dermatology residency, I developed a keen interest in how hair cosmetic issues intermingle with the medical issues of hair damage and loss. Finally, now as a practicing dermatologist functioning as a consultant to industry, I have insight into how the cosmetic, medical, and product development issues surrounding hair have created a large industry.

It is this synthesis of knowledge and expertise that I hope to share in this text. I have chosen to accomplish this goal through the use of words and pictures, both of which are equally important in obtaining a medical understanding of hair. The book attempts to seamlessly combine text and images to leave the reader with a fund of knowledge regarding the nonliving fibrillar keratin attached to our scalp, known as hair.

1 Hair physiology

HAIR STRUCTURE AND EMBRYOLOGY

Hair contributes significantly to the visual image of both males and females of all ages. Every visible major body surface is covered with some type of hair, providing the creation of endless opportunities for cosmetic adornment. Hair is nonliving, yet is immersed in a cycle of constant renewal and shedding. Unlike vital organs, such as the heart, liver, or kidneys, where limited cellular renewal can occur, hair growth occurs at the amazing rate of 0.35 mm/day allowing the removal of old, damaged hair that is readily replaced with new regrowth.[1] Hair is the only body structure that is completely renewable without scarring, as long as the follicle remains a functioning unit. For this reason, the hair can be subjected to insults that could not be sustained by any other body organ. This constant renewal also means that induced cosmetic alterations in shape, color, or texture are temporary until the chemically altered hair is sloughed or trimmed[2] (Figure 1.1).

The hair is a body structure readily accessible for scientific observation, yet much remains to be understood regarding its growth and regulation. The first dermatologist to encourage study of the hair was P.G. Unna of Hamburg in 1876.[3] One of Unna's students, Martin Engman (Professor of Dermatology, Washington University, St Louis), became interested in the embryology and development of the hair follicle. His work was furthered by C.H. Danforth, Mildred Trotter, and L.D. Cady, who published the foundation work on hair formation in 1925.[4]

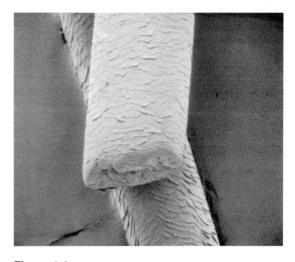

Figure 1.1
The appearance of the cut end of a solitary hair shaft.

Further works on the development of the hair follicle continued with Sengel (1976),[6] and Spearman (1977).[7,8] From this discussion, it should be apparent that hair research is a relatively modern interest, even though concerns about hair growth and loss date back to antiquity.

The hair follicle number that is present at birth remains constant throughout youth, slowly decreasing with age. Hair follicles are formed early in development of the fetus with eyebrow, upper lip, and chin follicles present at week 9 and the full complement of follicles present by week 22 (Figure 1.2). At this time, the total body number of 5 million follicles is present with 1 million on the head, of which 100,000 are on the scalp.[9] No additional follicles are formed during life. As body size increases, the number of hair follicles per unit area decreases. This gradual decrease is demonstrated in Table 1.1.[10]

The hair grows from follicles, which resemble stocking-like invaginations of the epithelium enclosing an area of dermis, known as the dermal papillae. The area of active cell division, the living area of the hair, is formed around the dermal papillae and is known as the bulb where cell division occurs every 23–72 hours.[11] The follicles slope into

Table 1.1 Scalp hair density variation with age

Age	Scalp hair density (per square centimeter)
Newborn	1135
One year	795
30 years	615

the dermis at varying angles, depending on body location and individual variation, and reside at varying levels between the lower dermis and the subcutaneous fat. In general, larger hairs have more deeply placed follicles than finer hairs.[12] An arrector pili muscle attaches to the midsection of the follicle wall and ends at the junction between the epidermis and dermis. In some body areas, a sebaceous gland and an apocrine gland attach above the muscle and open into the follicle. The point at which the arrector pili muscle attaches is known as the hair 'bulge' and is considered to be the site where new matrix cells are formed and the hair growth cycle is initiated (Figure 1.3). It takes approximately 3 weeks for a newly formed hair to appear at the scalp surface.

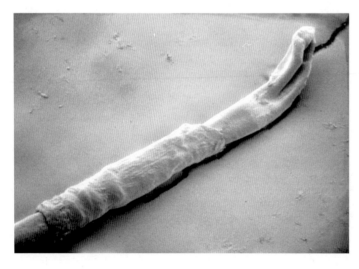

Figure 1.2
The appearance of the entire hair extracted intact from the follicle.

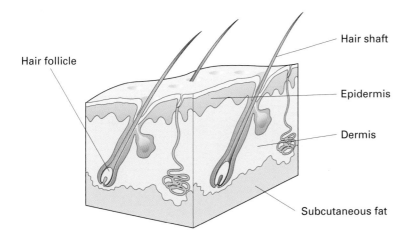

Hair follicle

Hair shaft

Epidermis

Dermis

Subcutaneous fat

Figure 1.3
The anatomy of the hair follicle in the skin.

The sebaceous gland is intimately associated with each and every hair shaft. Sebum is important to the maintenance of the grown hair shaft, as it functions as a natural conditioning agent removing static electricity and imparting shine to newly grown hair. Approximately 400–900 sebaceous glands per square centimeter are located on the scalp and represent the largest glands on the body.[13] Sebum, composed of free fatty acids and neutral fats, is produced in increased amounts after puberty in males and females and abundantly coats the hair shaft in youth. With advancing age, sebum production declines in the female with a less significant decrease in males. This leads us to the next topic of discussion, which is the hair growth cycle.

HAIR GROWTH CYCLE

Hair growth occurs on a cyclic basis with periods of growth, impending dormancy, and total dormancy occurring with clock-like accuracy. Each hair grows to a finite length depending upon predetermined genetic factors and age.[14–16] The growth phase, known

as anagen, lasts approximately 1000 days and the transitional phase, or catagen, about 2 weeks.[17] The resting phase, or telogen, lasts approximately 100 days (Table 1.2). Scalp hair is characterized by a relatively long anagen and a relatively short telogen with a ratio of anagen to telogen hairs of 90 to 10[18] (Figure 1.4). Only 1% or less of the follicles are in catagen at any given time. Thus, the healthy individual loses 100 hairs per day. It is estimated that each follicle completes this cycle 10–20 times over a life-time, but the activity of each follicle is independent.

The mechanism signaling the progression from one phase to the next is unknown, but

Table 1.2 Hair growth cycle

Hair growth phase	Duration of growth phase
Anagen (active growth)	1000 days
Catagen (pending dormancy)	14 days
Telogen (dormancy)	100 days

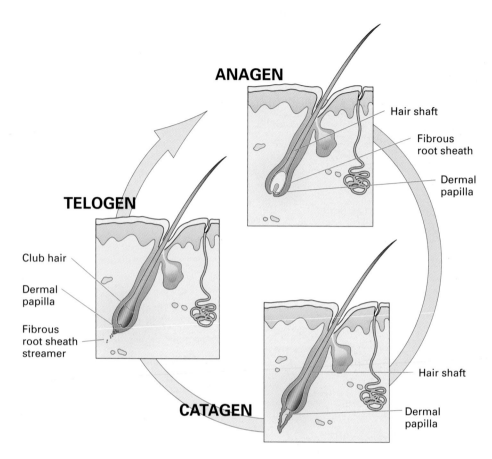

Figure 1.4
The appearance of the hair shaft and follicle at each of the stages of growth.

the duration of anagen determines the maximum length to which the hair can be grown. Hair growth can be affected by physical factors (severe illness, surgery, weight change, pregnancy, hormonal alterations, thyroid anomalies, dermatologic disease) and emotional factors, but is unaffected by physical alterations limited to the hair shaft (shaving, curling, combing, dyeing, etc.). Plucking of the hairs from resting follicles can stimulate growth, but the composition of the hair shaft remains the same, as discussed below.[19]

HAIR COMPOSITION

Hair is a nonliving structure basically formed of protein (Figure 1.5).[20–22] Specifically, it is composed of keratin, which is formed from insoluble cystine-containing helicoidal protein complexes. The hair is made up of an amorphous matrix high in sulfur proteins in which the keratin fibers are embedded.[23] These protein complexes, which form 65–95% of the hair by weight, are extraordinarily resistant to degradation and are thus

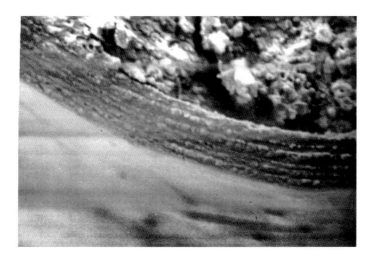

Figure 1.5
Cross-section through hair showing the structure of the cuticle and cortex layers.

termed hard keratins, as opposed to the soft keratins that compose the skin.[24] Under x-ray crystallography, the hair fiber helix has an alpha diffraction pattern, which changes to a beta diffraction pattern as the hair is stretched and the helix is pulled into a straight chain.

Each hair shaft is composed of a variety of layers, which are formed from closely attached keratinized fusiform cells arranged to form a cohesive fiber (Figure 1.6).[25] The greatest mass of the hair shaft is the central cortex, with some shafts also possessing a medulla. The cortex consists of closely packed spindle-shaped cells with their boundaries separated by a narrow gap, which contains a proteinaceous intercellular lamella thought to cement the cells together.[26] It is this structural organization of the cortex that provides mechanical strength to the hair shaft.

The cortex in turn surrounds the medulla, which is formed from a protein known as trichohyalin (Figure 1.7). The function of the medulla remains unknown; however, it contains glycogen and melanosomes. In older individuals, the medulla cells appear to dehydrate and air-filled spaces are left behind in place of a functional medulla.[27] In general, larger diameter hairs, such as those located on the scalp, are more likely to contain a medulla than finer body hairs.[28]

Surrounding the cortex is a protective layer of overlapping, keratinized scales known as the cuticle, which can account for up to 10% of the hair fiber by weight.[29,30] The cuticle free edges are directed outward with

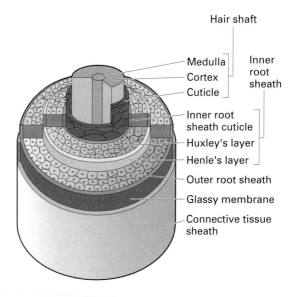

Figure 1.6
The layers of the hair shaft.

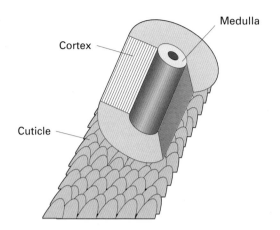

Figure 1.7
The organization of the cuticle, cortex, and medulla.

the proximal edges resting against the cortex (Figure 1.8).[31] The cuticular scales are arranged much like roofing shingles to provide five to ten overlapping cell layers, each 350–450 nm thick, to protect the hair shaft along its entire length. The cell structure of the cuticle is composed of three major layers: the A-layer, the exocuticle, and the endocuticle. It is the clear A-layer, which is high in sulfur-containing proteins, that protects the hair from chemical, physical, and environmental insults.[32] A healthy hair shaft is characterized by an intact, well-organized cuticle (Figure 1.9). It is this unusual structure of the hair shaft that provides for the unique physical properties of hair.[33]

HAIR PHYSICAL PROPERTIES

The physical properties of the hair shaft are related to its geometric shape and the organization of its constituents.[34] As mentioned previously, the cortex is largely responsible for the strength of the hair shaft, but an intact cuticle is necessary to resist externally applied mechanical stresses. The most common mechanical stress a hair must withstand is stretching, due to the trauma of grooming. This requires that the hair possess elastic properties, providing for stretch deformation followed by a return to a normal configuration. Hair can be stretched to 30% of its original length in water and experience no damage, but irreversible changes occur when hairs are stretched to between 30% and 70% of their

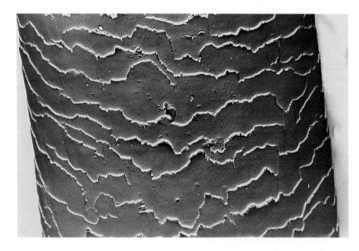

Figure 1.8
Cuticle cross-section viewed under electron microscopy.

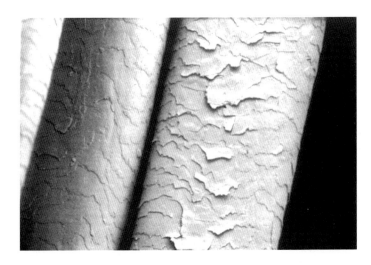

Figure 1.9
Uplifted cuticle scales indicative of hair shaft damage.

original length. Stretching to 80% of original length generally results in hair shaft fracture.[35]

In addition to undergoing stretch deformation, the hair shaft must also withstand repeated wetting and drying experienced as part of the hair cleansing process. It is water within the hair shaft that provides for optimal elasticity, but water can also be absorbed externally. The porosity of the hair shaft is about 20%, allowing a weight increase of 12–18% when soaked in water. The absorption rate is very rapid, with 75% of the maximum absorbable water entering the hair˝ shaft within 4 minutes.[36] Water absorption causes hair shaft swelling, which is the first step in cosmetic chemical treatments to be discussed in Chapters 6 and 7. Wetting and subsequent drying of the hair shaft in a predetermined position is also basic to hair styling, discussed in Chapter 4.

Another important physical characteristic of hair is the interaction between adjacent hair shafts in the form of friction. It has been shown that wet straight hair possesses higher combing friction than dry straight hair. This is an interesting observation leading to the idea that hair should not be combed when wet to avoid stretching the

hair shafts to the brittle breaking point.[37] Another interaction between the hair shafts is the production of static electricity. Static electricity preferentially affects dry hair since the ions are poorly conducted down the hair shaft. This is in contrast to wet hair, which is an excellent conductor due to the presence of water. Static electricity creates a hair grooming problem, since the hair shafts repel one another creating 'flyaway' hair that sticks away from the scalp. The static electricity between hair shafts can be reduced by decreasing hair friction, combing hair under cooler conditions, or decreasing the resistance of hair fibers by increasing hair moisture. These concepts will be revised when we consider hair grooming in Chapter 4.

The last issue to consider with regard to the physical characteristics of hair is hair shape. The shape of the hair is determined by its cross-sectional appearance (Figure 1.10). Caucasoid hair has an elliptical cross-section accounting for a slight curl, while Mongoloid hair has a circular cross-section leading to straight hair[38] (Figures 1.11 and 1.12). Negroid hair is identical to Caucasoid and Mongoloid hair in its amino acid content, but has a slightly larger diameter, lower

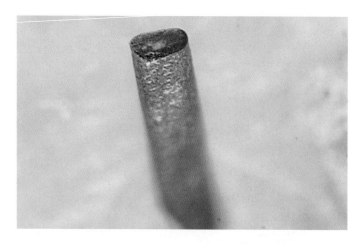

Figure 1.10
Cross-sectional electron microscopic appearance of a straight round hair shaft demonstrating the cortex and cuticle layers.

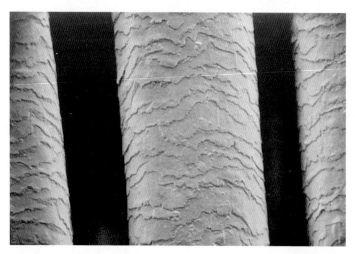

Figure 1.11
Caucasian hair shaft shape.

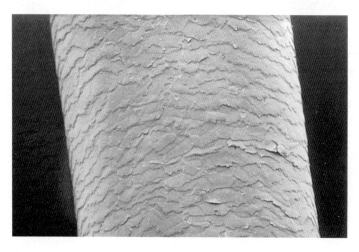

Figure 1.12
Asian hair shaft shape.

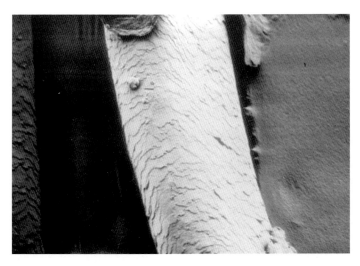

Figure 1.13
African-American hair shaft shape.

water content and, most importantly, a flattened elliptical cross-sectional shape[39] (Figure 1.13). It is the asymmetry of this cross-section that accounts for the irregular kinky appearance of Black hair[40] (Figure 1.14). Hair that is wavy or loosely kinked has a cross-sectional shape in between a circle and flattened ellipse (Figure 1.15).

The cross-sectional shape of the hair fiber accounts for more than the degree of curl, it also determines the amount of shine and the ability of sebum to coat the hair shaft.[41] Straight hair possesses more shine than kinky hair due to its smooth surface, allowing maximum light reflection and ease of sebum movement from the scalp down the hair shaft (Figure 1.16). The irregularly kinked hair shafts appear duller, even though they may have an intact cuticle, due to rough surface and difficulty encountered in sebum transport from the scalp, even though Black hair tends to produce more sebum (Figure 1.17).

The shape of the hair shaft also determines grooming ease. Straight hair is the easiest to groom, since combing friction is

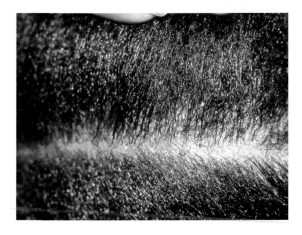

Figure 1.14
The appearance of African-American hair is due to the irregular cross-sectional shape.

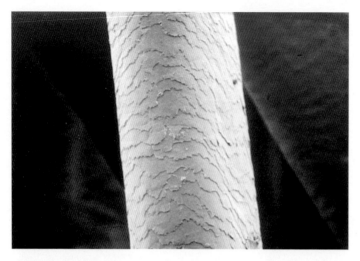

Figure 1.15
Curly Caucasian hair shaft shape.

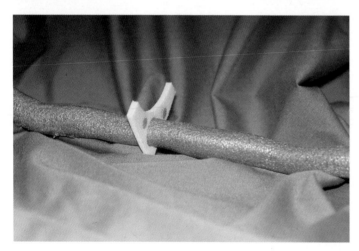

Figure 1.16
The yellow triangle represents sebum traversing a straight hair shaft.

low and the hair is easy to arrange in a fashionable style. Kinky hair, on the other hand, demonstrates increased grooming friction, resulting in increased hair shaft breakage. Kinky hair also does not easily conform to a predetermined hair style, unless the shafts are short. These issues where hair physical properties determine the ability to style hair will be revisited later in Chapter 3.

HAIR LOSS IN MEN AND WOMEN

Hair loss is a common reason for male and female patients to consult the dermatologist. It is easy for the patient to state that their hair is falling out, but far more difficult for the physician to determine the exact cause and provide effective treatment. Hair

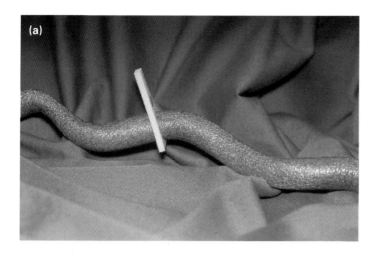

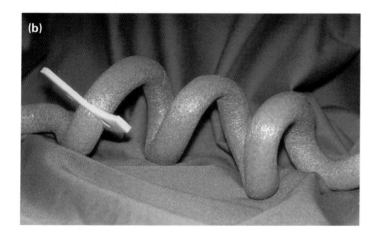

Figure 1.17
The yellow triangle represents sebum traveling down a wavy hair with more difficulty (a) and down a kinky hair shaft with even more difficulty (b).

can be shed for many reasons, some medical and some cosmetic. This section will deal with an abbreviated approach to addressing the patient with medical hair loss (Figure 1.18).

Generally, patients state that their usually thick, shiny and manageable hair has become thin and difficult to style. If this is the dermatologist's first consultation with the patient, verifying the degree of hair loss is difficult. It is estimated that an individual must lose approximately 50% of their hair before an unacquainted observer can examine the scalp and note a reduction in hair shaft number. In the hair cosmetics industry, there is an established minimum number of hair shafts that are considered necessary to present the perception of a full head of hair (Table 1.3). This type of information is used in the manufacture of natural-looking hairpieces and wigs. In general, red hair requires fewer shafts than blond hair to appear full,

Figure 1.18
Patient with hair thinning due to
follicular degeneration syndrome.

**Table 1.3 Number of hair shafts required
for the appearance of hair fullness by hair
color**

Hair color	Scalp hair shaft number
Blond	140,000
Brown	110,000
Black	108,000
Red	90,000

this section describes my approach to the patient with diffuse, nonscarring hair loss. Pertinent questions are asked in logical order to arrive correctly at a diagnosis to initiate appropriate treatment (Box 1.1). Scarring causes of hair loss are beyond the realm of this text.[41]

1. Is the hair loss due to external or internal causation?
The initial step in determining the type of hair loss experienced by the patient is to determine whether the loss is due to internal causes that are medically treatable or external causes that are cosmetically treatable. This can easily be determined by examining the hair bulb under the microscope. The hair bulb is the remnants of the structures of the

since red hair shafts have the thickest diameter while blond hair shafts are the thinnest (Figure 1.19).

Hair loss is a complex problem mediated by internal and external factors. The rest of

---

Box 1.1 Hair loss diagnosis algorithm

1. Is the hair loss due to external or internal causation?
    Examine shed hair bulb under microscope for hair bulb morphology.
2. What is the magnitude of the hair loss?
    Gently perform 10 hair clump pulls randomly throughout scalp.
3. Is hair breakage occurring?
    Have patient collect 4 consecutive days of hair loss and place each day's loss in a separate plastic bag, noting if the hair was shampooed on that day on the outside of the bag.
4. Is there a treatable medical cause?
    Evaluate past medical history and review of systems.

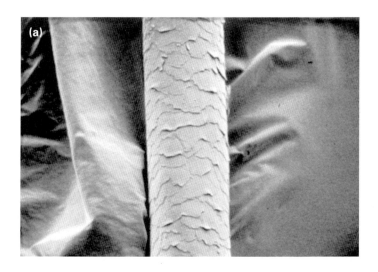

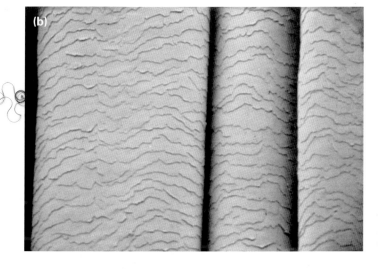

Figure 1.19
Thin Caucasian hair shaft appearance (a) versus a thick Caucasian hair shaft (b).

hair follicle, which appear as a clear attachment to the proximal end of the hair shaft.

Hairs can be shed during two phases of growth, anagen and telogen. Anagen hairs have an elongated bulb while telogen hairs have a clubbed bulb. Anagen is the growth phase of the hair follicle. Hairs shed prematurely during this phase are shed as a result of some severe internal health issue and possess an elongated tubular bulb. This type of hair loss is known as anagen effluvium. Normally, hairs are shed during the telogen or resting phase of the hair follicle. Hairs are shed during telogen to allow the follicle to rest prior to initiating growth of a new hair and the return of the anagen phase. Telogen hairs possess a club-shaped proximal end. If the body has prematurely placed many hair follicles into the resting phase, the condition is known as telogen effluvium.

2. What is the magnitude of the hair loss?

Hair loss can be easily distinguished from hair breakage by performing 10 hair pulls over various areas of the scalp. The hair pull is performed by grasping the hair shaft close to the scalp with the fingers and firmly pulling over the length of the shaft. Removed hairs are examined for the presence and formation of the bulb. If more than six hairs are removed per pull, excessive hair loss is present. This procedure also provides an opportunity to determine if any scalp disease is present that might be contributing to the hair loss.

However, hair pulls in the office can be misleading, especially if the patient has shampooed prior to being examined and has removed the loose or broken hairs. Questioning of the patient as to the magnitude of hair loss may also be misleading, since most are not aware that a normal individual may lose approximately100 hairs per day. If grooming of the hair is infrequent, shampooing may yield up to 200 or more lost hairs.

3. Is hair breakage occurring?

Hair breakage occurs as a result of weakness in the structure of the hair shaft. Information about the magnitude of hair breakage can best be obtained by having the patient collect all hair lost for 4 consecutive days and place each day's loss in a separate plastic bag, noting the days when shampooing was performed. The hair should be brushed or combed over the sink and the hair collected from the sink and also from the brush or comb. Hairs should also be removed from the drain following shampooing. The dermatologist can examine each day's loss, noting both amount and presence or absence of

the hair bulb to determine in which growth phase the hairs were shed and also if hair breakage has occurred.

Hair breakage can result from improper grooming practices, the topic of discussion in Chapter 7. However, abnormally formed hair shafts, found sporadically or in association with genodermatoses (trichoschisis, trichorrhexis invaginata, pili torti, monilethrix, and trichorrhexis nodosa), can also result in decreased hair shaft strength and subsequent breakage. Examination of several plucked hairs under the microscope is necessary to insure normal hair structure. This topic is discussed more fully in the next section.

4. Is there a treatable medical cause?

If more than 100–125 hairs are lost per day, and it has been determined that normally formed hairs are being shed diffusely from a nonscarred scalp with an intact bulb, anagen effluvium, telogen effluvium, and other medically induced causes must be considered. Anagen effluvium is generally due to internally administered medications, such as chemotherapy agents, that act as cell poisons and disrupt the growing hair follicle. Telogen effluvium, on the other hand, is due to an increased number of hair follicles prematurely exiting the anagen phase or hair cycle synchronization.[42] Premature anagen exit can be due to medications, such as coumarin or heparin, while hair cycle synchronization occurs during pregnancy and with oral contraceptive use.

There are several medical causes of hair loss, which require treatment prior to hair regrowth. These are summarized in Box 1.2. Most of these considerations can be addressed via a review of systems and basic laboratory tests. Anemia, thyroid abnormalities and many illnesses can be evaluated by obtaining a complete blood count with differential, thyroid panel, and chemistry panel to include liver function

---

Box 1.2 Medical causes of alopecia

1. Physical stress: surgery, illness (acute or chronic), anemia, lack of sleep
2. Emotional stress: psychiatric illness, death of family member, job loss, marital difficulties
3. Diet considerations: rapid weight loss or gain, unusual dieting habits, vegetarian, protein intake failure, prolonged fasting
4. Hormonal causes: postpartum, oral contraceptives, menopause, insufficient hormone supplementation, ingestion of testosterone-containing hormone supplements
5. Endocrinopathy: hypothyroidism, hyperthyroidism, hypoparathyroidism, hyperparathyroidism
6. Oral medications:
   a. blood thinning agents: heparin, coumarin
   b. retinoids: high dose vitamin A, isotretinoin, etretinate
   c. antihypertensive agents: propranolol, captopril
   d. miscellaneous: quinacrine, allopurinol, lithium carbonate, thiouracil compounds

---

studies. If deemed clinically necessary, an antinuclear antibody (ANA) can also be obtained to rule out any collagen vascular diseases. A complete history can determine the nature of any severe physical or emotional stress and document the ingestion of prescription or over-the-counter medications or vitamin supplements.

The three most common medical causes of female hair loss in a dermatology practice are the influences of physical stress, emotional stress, diet considerations, and hormonal difficulties. These are addressed in more detail below.

a. Is the patient experiencing physical or emotional stress?

Physical and emotional stress divert the body's energies away from nonlife-sustaining activities, such as growing hair, to maintenance of the organs vital for survival, such as the heart, lungs, kidneys, liver, etc. Typically, it will take the body 6–9 months to reinitiate cosmetically visible hair growth after surgery, febrile illness, or severe emo-

tional stress. For this reason, the physician should take a history of the patient's activities for at least the past year. In many cases, a 3-month delay is present between the actual event and the patient's onset of hair loss. Furthermore, there may be another 3-month delay prior to the return of noticeable hair regrowth. Thus, the total hair loss and regrowth cycle can last 6 months, 9 months, or possibly longer. This timetable can be used to help the patient understand when hair regrowth can be expected.

b. Is there a dietary cause for the hair loss?

Hair loss due to rapid weight change or unusual dietary intake is not uncommon. Yo-yo dieting among young people is a frequent cause of hair loss where the body enters periods of starvation, during which time energy is diverted away from hair growth. The rapid fluctuations in weight may precipitate continuous hair loss, since the body never achieves a 3-month period of stability when hair can regrow. These rapid fluctuations in weight are also seen in young

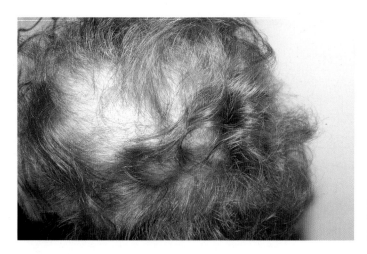

Figure 1.20
The typical pattern of female pattern hair loss.

persons with eating disorders such as anorexia nervosa and bulemia.

Fad dieting may also be a problem when the diet is intentionally unbalanced to promote weight loss. Such diets include eating only grapefruit, which will result in weight loss, but also hair loss, due to the inadequate protein intake. Another fad diet is eating foods that are rich in protein while avoiding fruits, vegetables, and carbohydrates to put the body into a state of ketosis to decrease the appetite. Prolonged ketosis will also result in hair loss. It is best if the dieting can be done in a gradual manner, losing no more than half a pound weekly, while maintaining a balanced intake of protein and nutrients. This type of weight loss will spare the patient unnecessary hair loss.

b. Are hormonal abnormalities precipitating hair loss?
Hormonal causes of hair loss deserve special attention in the female patient. Many women do not realize that hair loss can present postpartum or following discontinuation of oral contraceptives. It is important to remind the female patient that hair loss may be delayed by 3 months following a hormonal status change and another 3–6 months may be required for regrowth to be fully appreciated.

Perimenopausal and menopausal women with decreased ovarian estrogen production may also experience diffuse hair thinning, generally more prominent over the top of the head with bitemporal recession. A thin strip of hair at the anterior hairline is usually spared (Figure 1.20). Obtaining a follicle-stimulating hormone (FSH) level can be helping in determining if the patient is in menopause. However, many women will begin to experience significant hair loss, even though the FSH level is within the normal range. In this case, it is still advantageous to begin estrogen hormone replacement therapy, provided that there are other symptoms of menopause, such as irregular menses, hot flashes, night sweats, fatigue, depression, mood swings, crying spells, etc. Early hormone replacement therapy can prevent further loss, but has not been shown to promote regrowth. Other treatments such as topical minoxidil or an off-label trial of oral finasteride may be indicated.[43]

Lastly, it is important to rule out any hormonal abnormalities in the female patient. Inquiring as to the regularity of menses and the presence of infertility problems can uncover ovarian hormonal failure or the presence of excess endogenous androgens. Questions should also be directed as to whether the patient is ingesting oral steroids with androgenic effects. If necessary, hormone levels such as a free testosterone and dehydroepiandrosterone sulfate (DHEA-S) can be drawn and an endocrinologic evaluation initiated.[44] Some women may also be ingesting a hormone replacement therapy that includes testosterone. It is felt that testosterone is necessary to prevent vaginal dryness and increase libido in some women with sexual dysfunction. Unfortunately, this testosterone supplementation may cause the onset of female pattern hair loss in susceptible women. A more detailed discussion of hormonally induced hair loss is beyond the scope of this text.[45,46]

HAIR SHAFT STRUCTURAL ABNORMALITIES

There are a number of internal diseases and external cosmetic causes that contribute to hair shaft structural abnormalities. These hair shaft abnormalities lead to hair shaft weakness resulting in hairs shed without an intact hair bulb and broken hairs. Box 1.3 contains the technical terms used to

---

Box 1.3 Structural hair shaft abnormalities

INTRINSIC ABNORMALITIES
1. Trichoschisis – A clean, transverse fracture across the hair shaft through both cuticle and cortex. Congenital forms seen in trichothiodystrophy characterized by hair with an abnormally low sulfur content.
2. Trichorrhexis invaginata – A nodular expansion of the hair shaft in which a ball in socket joint is formed, also known as bamboo hair. Congenital forms seen in Netherton's syndrome.
3. Pili torti – A flattened hair shaft that is twisted through 180 degrees on its own axis.
4. Monilethrix – elliptical nodal swellings along the hair shaft with intervening, tapering constrictions that are nonmedullated.

EXTRINSIC ABNORMALITIES
1. Trichoptilosis – A longitudinal splitting or fraying of the distal end of the hair shaft, also known as split ends.
3. Trichonodosis – Knotting of the hair shaft.

INTRINSIC OR EXTRINSIC ABNORMALITIES
1. Trichorrhexis nodosa – Small, beaded swellings associated with a loss of the cuticle.
Congenital forms seen in argininosuccinic aciduria and Menke's disease, but may also be due to cosmetic hair shaft manipulation.

describe hair shaft abnormalities and definitions of the terms.[47] Trichoschisis, trichorrhexis invaginata, pili torti, and monilethrix are all abnormalities intrinsic to the hair shaft.[48] Trichoptilosis and trichonodosis may be due to cosmetic manipulation of the hair. Trichorrhexis nodosa may be due to intrinsic abnormalities or cosmetic manipulation. All of these conditions predispose the hair to breakage, which can become magnified by extensive grooming, chemical waving procedures or permanent dyeing. The topic of hair grooming is considered in the next chapter.

REFERENCES

1. Myers RJ, Hamilton JB. Regeneration and rate of growth of hair in man. *Ann N Y Acad Sci* 1951;**53**:862.

2. Herman S. Hair 101: understanding the architecture of a hair shaft can help in formulating treatment products. *GCI* 2001;14–16.

3. Unna PG. Beitrage zur histologie und entwicklengsgeschichte der menschlichen oberhat und ihrer anhangsgebilde. *Arch fur microscopisch Anatomie und Entwicklungsmach* 1876;**12**:665.

4. Danforth CH. Hair with special reference to hypertrichosis. *AMA Archives of Dermatology and Syphilogy* 1925;**11**:494.

5. Sengel P. *Morphogenesis of skin*. Cambridge: Cambridge University Press, 1976.

6. Spearman RIC. Hair follicle development, cyclical changes and hair form. In: Jarrett A, ed. *The hair follicle*. London: Academic Press, 1977:1268.

7. Rook A, Dawber R. *Diseases of the hair and scalp*. Oxford: Blackwell Scientific Publications, 1982:5–6.

8. Dawber R, Van Neste D. *Hair and scalp disorders*. Philadelphia: J.B. Lippincott Company, 1995:4.

9. Giacometti L. The anatomy of the human scalp. In: Montagna W, Dobson RL, eds. *Advances in biology of skin*, Vol. IX, *Hair growth*. Oxford: Pergamon Press, 1969:97.

10. Van Scott EJ, Ekel TM, Auerbach R. Determinants of rate and kinetics of cell division in scalp hair. *J Invest Dermatol* 1963;**41**:269.

11. Durward A, Rudall KM. The vascularity and patterns of growth of hair follicles. In: Montagna W, Ellis RA, eds. *The biology of hair growth*. New York: Academic Press, 1958:189.

12. Benfenati A, Brillanti F. Sulla distribuziona della ghiandole sebacee nella cute del corpo umano. *Arch Ital Dermatol Sifilogr Venereol* 1939;**15**:33–42.

13. Kligman AM. The human hair cycle. *J Invest Dermatol* 1959;**33**:307.

14. Robbins C, Robbins M. Scalp hair length. I. Hair length in Florida theme parks: an approximation of hair length in the United States of America. *J Cosmet Sci* 2003;**54**:53–62.

15. Robbins C, Robbins M. Scalp hair length. II. Estimating the percentage of adults in the USA and larger populations by hair length. *J Cosmet Sci* 2003;**54**:367–78.

16. Orentreich N. Scalp hair regeneration in man. In: Montagna W, Dobson RL, eds. *Advances in biology of skin*, Vol. IX, *Hair growth*. Oxford: Pergamon Press, 1969:99.

17. Witzel M, Braun-Falco O. Uber den haarwurzelstatus am menschlichen capillitium unter physiologischen bedingungen. *Archiv fur Klinische und Experimentelle Dermatologie* 1963;**216**:221.

18. Dawber R, Van Neste D. *Hair and scalp disorders*. Philadelphia: J.B. Lippincott, 1995:15.

19. Wolfram L. Human hair: a unique physico-chemical composite. *J Am Acad Dermatol* 2003;**48** (Suppl): S106–S114.

20. Rossi A, Barbieri L, Pistola G, Bonaccorsi P, Calvieri S. Hair and nail structure and function. *J Appl Cosmetol* 2003;**21**:1–8.

21. Ebina S, Yamaki M. Nucleic acid is a major water-extractable acidic macromolecule of human scalp hair. *J Cosmet Sci* 1999;**50**:297–305.

22. Smith J. Use of atomic force microscopy for high-resolution non-invasive structural studies of human hair. *J Soc Cosmet Chem* 1997;**48**:199–208.

23. Robbins CR. *Chemical and physical behavior of the hair*. New York: Van Nostrand-Reinhold, 1979:7.

24. Odland GF. Structure of the skin. In: Goldsmith LA, ed. *Physiology, biochemistry, and molecular biology of the skin*, 2nd edn. Oxford: Oxford University Press, 1991:46.

25. Braun-Falco O. The fine structure of the anagen hair follicle of the mouse. In: Montagna W, Dobson RL, eds. *Advances in biology of skin*, Vol. IX, *Hair growth*. Oxford: Pergamon Press, 1969: chapter 29.

26. Nagase S, Shibuichi S, Ando K, Kariya E, Satoh N. Influence of internal structures on hair appearance. I. Light scattering from the porous structure of the medulla of human hair. *J Cosmet Sci* 2002;**53**:89–100.

27. Marhle G, Orfanos GE. The spongious keratin and the medullary substance of human scalp hair. *Archiv fur Dermatologische Forschung* 1971;**241**:305.

28. Wolfram LJ, Lindemann MKO. Some observations on the hair cuticle. *J Soc Cosmet Chem* 1971;**22**:839.

29. Atsuta C, Fukumashi A, Fukuda M. Mechanism of isolation of human hair cuticle with KOH/1-butanol solutions. *J Soc Cosmet Chem* 1995;**46**:281–90.

30. Swift J. Human hair cuticle: biologically conspired to the owner's advantage. *J Cosmet Sci* 1999;**50**:23–47.

31. Swift JA. The histology of keratin fibres. In: Asquith RA, ed. *Chemistry of natural protein fibres*. London: Wiley, 1977: chapter 3.

32. Nagase S, Satoh N, Nakamura K. Influence of internal structure of hair fiber on hair appearance. II. Consideration of the visual perception mechanism of hair appearance. *J Cosmet Sci* 2002;**53**:387–402.

33. Stocklassa B, Aranay-Vitores M, Nilsson G *et al*. Evaluation of a new X-ray fluorescent analysis technique for the creation of a Nordic hair database: elemental distributions within the root and the virgin segment of hair fibers. *J Cosmet Sci* 2001;**52**:297–311.

34. Alexander P, Hudson PF, Earland C. *Wool: its chemistry and physics*, 2nd edn. London: Chapman & Hall, 1963.

35. Rook A, Dawber R. *Diseases of the hair and scalp*. Oxford: Blackwell Scientific Publications, 1982:36–7.

36. Meredith R, Hearle J. *Physical methods of investigating textiles*. New York: Interscience, 1959.

37. Lindelof B, Forslind B, Hedblad M *et al*. Human hair form: morphology revealed by light and scanning electron microscopy and computer-aided three-dimensional reconstruction. *Arch Dermatol* 1988;**124**:1359–63.

38. Brooks G, Lewis A. Treatment regimes for styled Black hair. *Cosmet Toilet* 1983;**98**:59–68.

39. Johnson BA. Requirements in cosmetics for black skin. *Dermatol Clin* 1988;**6**:409–92.

40. Bergfeld WF. Scarring alopecia. In: Roenigk RR, Roenigk HR, eds. *Dermatologic surgery, principles and practice*. New York: Marcel Dekker, 1989:759–79.

41. Headington JT. Telogen effluvium. *Arch Dermatol* 1993;**129**:356–63.

42. Olsen EA, DeLong ER, Weiner MS. Safe response study of topical minoxidil in male pattern baldness. *J Am Acad Dermatol* 1986;**15**:30–7.

43. Redmond GP, Bergfeld WF. Diagnostic approach to androgen disorders in women. *Cleve Clin J Med* 1990;**57**:423–32.

44. Sperling LC, Heimer WL. Androgen biology as a basis for the diagnosis and treatment of androgenic disorders in women. I. *J Am Acad Dermatol* 1993;**28**:669–83.

45. Sperling LC, Heimer WL. Androgen biology as a basis for the diagnosis and treatment of androgenic disorders in women. II. *J Am Acad Dermatol* 1993;**28**:901–16.

46. Whiting DA. Structural abnormalities of the hair shaft. *J Am Acad Dermatol* 1987;**16**:1–25.

47. Camacho-Martinez F, Ferrando J. Hair shaft dysplasias. *Int J Dermatol* 1988;**27**:71–80.

2 Hair grooming

SHAMPOOS

Shampoo is a cleanser designed to remove sebum, eccrine sweat, apocrine sweat, fungal elements, desquamated corneocytes, styling products, and environmental dirt from the scalp and hair[1] (Figures 2.1 and 2.2). The main purpose of a shampoo is to cleanse the scalp, but most patients would disagree, stating that the purpose of shampoo is to beautify the hair. This perception that a shampoo can impart cosmetic value to nonliving hair shafts has led to the tremendous plethora of shampoos on the market today.[2] This section delves into the formulation, efficacy, and variety of liquid mass-market shampoos.

Cleansing the hair is actually a complex task, since the average woman has 4–8 square meters of hair surface area to clean.[3] It is very easy to formulate a shampoo that will remove dirt, but hair that has had all the sebum removed is dull in appearance, coarse to the touch, subject to static electricity, and more difficult to style.[4] Traditional bar soaps are not recommended for hair

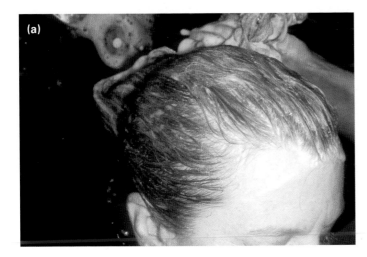

(a)

Figure 2.1
Proper shampooing technique in a female with long hair. (a) Hair and scalp are wetted and the liquid shampoo is distributed.

Figure 2.1 continued

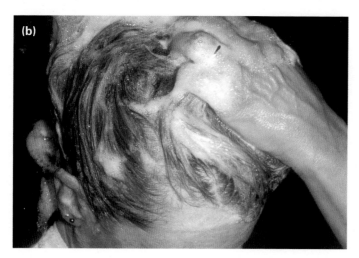

(b) Shampoo is foamed and massaged into the scalp.

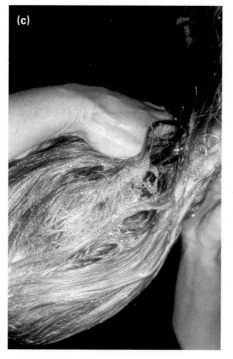

(c) Shampoo foam is distributed throughout the hair.

Figure 2.1 continued

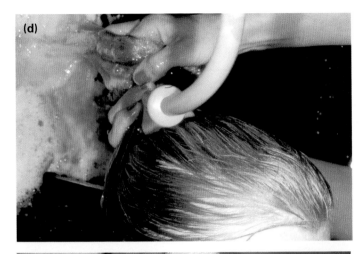

(d) Water is used to thoroughly rinse the hair and scalp.

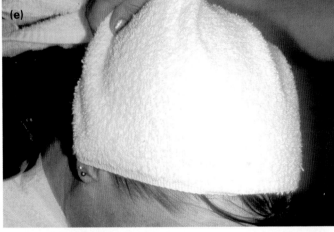

(e) Hair is towel-dried to absorb excess water.

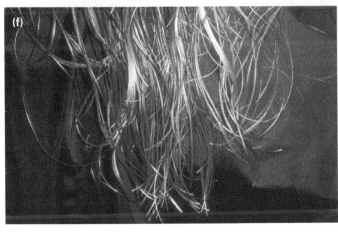

(f) Hair is detangled with a wide-toothed comb.

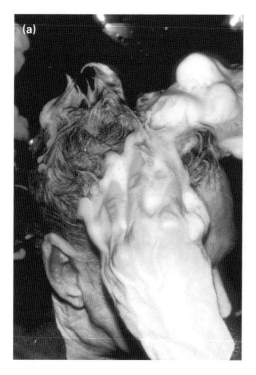

Figure 2.2
Proper shampooing technique in a male. (a) Hair
and scalp are wetted and the shampoo is foamed
and massaged into the scalp.

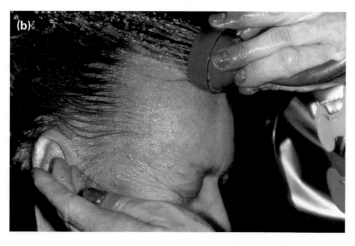

(b) Hair is rinsed with abundant
water.

Figure 2.2 continued

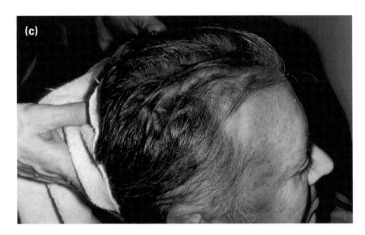

(c) Hair is towel-dried.

cleansing because they leave behind a soap scum when mixed with hard water that is difficult to rinse from the hair and scalp. This may be one of the aggravating factors for seborrheic dermatitis. Table 2.1 lists the general ingredient categories and their function in a basic shampoo formulation.[5] Each of these categories will be discussed in detail.

Table 2.1 Basic shampoo ingredient formulation and function

Ingredient	Function
1. Detergents	Functions to remove environment dirt, styling products, sebum, and skin scale from the hair and scalp
2. Foaming agents	This agent allows the shampoo to foam, since consumers equate cleansing with foaming even though the two are unrelated
3. Conditioners	Leave the hair soft and smooth after sebum removal by the detergent
4. Thickeners	Thicken the shampoo, since consumers feel that a thick shampoo works better than a thin shampoo
5. Opacifiers	Added to make a shampoo opaque as opposed to translucent for esthetic purposes unrelated to cleansing
6. Sequestering agents	Function to prevent soap scum from forming on the hair and scalp in the presence of hard water. The basic difference between a liquid shampoo and a bar cleanser
7. Fragrances	Added to give the shampoo a smell that is acceptable to the consumer
8. Preservatives	Prevent microbial and fungal contamination of the shampoo before and after opening
9. Specialty additives	Treatment ingredients or marketing aids added to impart other benefits to the shampoo besides hair and scalp cleansing

Shampoo detergents

Shampoos function by employing detergents, also known as surfactants, which are amphiphilic. This means that the detergent molecule possesses both lipophilic, or oil-attracting, and hydrophilic, or water-attracting, sites. The lipophilic site binds to sebum and oil-soluble dirt while the hydrophilic site binds to water, allowing removal of the sebum with water rinsing.[6] Box 2.1 lists the shampoo detergents currently available to the cosmetic chemist for use in shampoo formulations.[7]

Box 2.1 Shampoo detergents by chemical category

- Alkyl sulfates
- Alkyl ether sulfates
- Alpha-olefin sulfonates
- Paraffin sulfonates
- Isethionates
- Sarconsinates
- Taurides
- Acyl lactylates
- Sulfosuccinates
- Carboxylates
- Protein condensates
- Betaines
- Glycinates
- Amine oxides

Typically, several detergents are combined together to achieve the desired end result. For example, if the shampoo is intended for oily hair, detergents with strong sebum removal qualities are selected, conversely if the shampoo is intended for permanently waved or dyed hair, mild detergents are selected to reduce sebum removal. The art of shampoo formulation is selecting the right detergent combination to cleanse the scalp and beautify the hair simultaneously. The most commonly used shampoo detergents are listed in Box 2.2.

Box 2.2 The most common shampoo detergents

- Sodium laureth sulfate
- Sodium lauryl sulfate
- TEA lauryl sulfate
- Ammonium laureth sulfate
- Ammonium lauryl sulfate
- DEA lauryl sulfate
- Sodium olefin sulfonate

There are four basic categories of shampoo detergents: anionics, cationics, amphoterics, nonionics and natural surfactants (Table 2.2).[8] Each of these groups possesses different hair cleansing and conditioning qualities, which are combined to yield the final shampoo characteristics.

Anionic detergents

Anionic detergents are the most popular surfactants used in basic cleansing shampoos in the current market. They are named for their negatively charged hydrophilic polar group. Anionic detergents are derived from fatty alcohols and are exceptionally adept at removing sebum from the scalp and hair. Unfortunately, the esthetics of thoroughly cleaned hair are not well accepted by the consumer. Hair devoid of all sebum is harsh, rough, subject to static electricity, dull, and hard to detangle. There are several common detergents categorized within the anionic group:

1. Chemical class: lauryl sulfates
    Most shampoos designed to produce good hair cleansing will contain a lauryl

Table 2.2 Shampoo detergent characteristics

Surfactant type	Chemical class	Characteristics
Anionics	Lauryl sulfates, laureth sulfates, sarcosines, sulfosuccinates	Deep cleansing, may leave hair harsh
Cationics	Long-chain amino esters, ammonioesters	Poor cleansing, poor lather, impart softness and manageability
Nonionics	Polyoxyethylene fatty alcohols, polyoxyethylene sorbitol esters, alkanolamides	Mildest cleansing, impart manageability
Amphoterics	Betaines, sultaines, imidazolinium derivatives	Nonirritating to eyes, mild cleansing, impart manageability
Natural surfactants	Sarsaparilla, soapwort, soap bark, ivy, agave	Poor cleansing, excellent lather

sulfate as the second or third ingredient listed on the label, with water being the primary ingredient. The detergent listed first is the primary cleanser in highest concentration and the detergent listed second is the secondary cleanser designed to compliment the short-comings of the primary detergent. Examples of lauryl sulfate detergents include: sodium lauryl sulfate, triethanolamine lauryl sulfate, and ammonium lauryl sulfate. These ingredients are popular primary cleansers because they work well in both hard and soft water, produce rich foam, and are easily rinsed. They are excellent cleansers but hard on the hair, requiring careful selection of a secondary detergent and possible use of a conditioning agent as part of the shampoo formulation. Lauryl sulfates are commonly used in shampoos for oily hair.

2. Chemical class: laureth sulfates
    The laureth sulfates are one of the most commonly used primary detergents in general shampoos designed for normal to dry hair. They provide excellent cleansing, but leave the hair in good condition. Consumers like these detergents since they produce abundant foam, even though the amount of foam produced has nothing to do with adequate scalp and hair cleansing. Examples of detergents that fall into this chemical class as listed on the shampoo label are: sodium laureth sulfate, triethanolamine laureth sulfate, and ammonium laureth sulfate.

3. Chemical class: sarcosines
    The sarcosines are generally not used as primary detergents, since they do not excel at sebum removal. However, they are excellent conditioners and commonly used as the secondary or tertiary detergents, appearing second or third on the shampoo ingredient list. The sarcosines are used in conditioning shampoos and dry hair shampoos. Commonly employed detergents of this class include lauryl sarcosine and sodium lauryl sarcosinate.

4. Chemical class: sulfosuccinates
    The sulfosuccinates are strong detergents that are useful in removing sebum from oily hair. For this reason, they are a common secondary surfactant in oily hair shampoos. Commonly used

detergents from this class include di-sodium oleamine sulfosuccinate and sodium dioctyl sulfosuccinate.

Cationic detergents

The anionic detergents previously discussed are named for their negatively charged polar group, while the cationic detergents are named for their positively charged polar group. The cationic detergents are not nearly as popular in current shampoos as the anionic detergents because they are limited in their ability to remove sebum and do not produce the abundant lather desired by consumers. In addition, cationic detergents cannot be combined with anionic detergents, limiting their utility. Cationic detergents are primarily used in shampoos where minimal cleansing is desired, such as in daily shampoos designed for permanently dyed or chemically bleached hair. Cationic detergents are excellent at imparting softness and manageability to chemically damaged hair.[9]

Nonionic detergents

The nonionic detergents are the second most popular surfactant, behind the anionic detergents. They are named nonionic since they have no polar group. These detergents are the mildest of all surfactants and are used in combination with ionic surfactants as a secondary cleanser.[10] Examples of commonly used nonionic detergents include polyoxyethylene fatty alcohols, polyoxyethylene sorbitol esters, and alkanolamides.

Amphoteric detergents

The term amphoteric refers to substances that have both a negatively charged and a positively charged polar group. Thus, amphoteric detergents contain both an anionic and a cationic group, which allows them to behave as cationic detergents at lower pH values and as anionic detergents at higher pH values. These properties make amphoteric detergents quite unique. Within the amphoteric detergent category, there are several subgroups that include the betaines, sultaines, and imidazolinium derivatives. Amphoteric detergents, such as cocamidopropyl betaine and sodium lauraminopropionate, are found in baby shampoos. These detergents actually numb the tissues of the eyes, accounting for the nonstinging characteristics of baby shampoo. Amphoteric detergents are also used in shampoos for fine and chemically treated hair because they foam moderately well while leaving the hair manageable.

Natural detergents

The synthetic detergents previously discussed have largely replaced the natural detergents; some shampoos marketed as 'botanical' or 'natural' formulations may contain low levels of natural surfactants from plants such as sarsaparilla, soapwort, soap bark, and ivy agave. These natural saponins have excellent lathering capabilities, but are poor cleansers. Usually, they are combined with the other synthetic detergents previously discussed.[11] The synthetic detergents provide most of the hair and scalp cleansing while the botanicals are largely added for marketing purposes.

Foaming agents

One of the most important attributes of a shampoo from a consumer perspective is foaming ability. Consumers are convinced that a shampoo that foams poorly also cleans poorly. This is not the case. Most shampoos contain foaming agents to introduce gas bubbles into the water. The foam, also known as lather, is important since it functions to spread the detergent over the hair and scalp, but it does not participate in cleaning. It is true that a shampoo applied to dirty hair will not foam as much as the same shampoo applied to clean hair. This is due to the sebum inhibiting bubble formation. Thus, a shampoo will foam less on the first shampooing and more on the second shampooing.

Thickeners and opacifiers

Thickeners and opacifiers are added not to alter shampoo function, but to create esthetic appeal. Consumers believe that a thicker shampoo is more expensive and will produce better cleansing than a thin shampoo. This is not the case. Thicker shampoos are not richer shampoos, they simple have an agent added to increase viscosity. Opacifiers also play an esthetic role by making the clear shampoo opaque. Currently, opacifiers are added with light reflective properties to make the shampoo appear pearlescent. This appearance does not translate into any scalp or hair benefits.

Sequestering agents

Another important shampoo ingredient that does not participate in cleansing is the sequestering agent. Sequestering agents function to chelate magnesium and calcium ions, preventing the formation of insoluble soaps, known as 'scum.' Without sequestering agents, shampoos would leave a scum film on the hair making it appear dull. This same film can also form on the scalp, con-

tributing to itching and ultimately some of the symptoms of seborrheic dermatitis. For this reason, patients should be encouraged to use shampoo and not bar soap when cleansing the hair.

Conditioners

While the main intent of a shampoo is to cleanse the scalp and hair, overcleansed hair is not cosmetically acceptable. Hair that is completely devoid of sebum is harsh, difficult to style, and dull. Some persons wish to shampoo daily as a hygiene ritual, whether there has been adequate sebum production or not. Thus, shampoos formulated for dry, damaged, or chemically treated hair frequently contain a conditioner. The conditioner functions to impart manageability, gloss, and antistatic properties to the hair. These are usually fatty alcohols, fatty esters, vegetable oils, mineral oils, or humectants. Commonly used conditioning substances include hydrolyzed animal protein, glycerin, dimethicone, simethicone, polyvinylpyrrolidone, propylene glycol, and stearalkonium chloride.[12,13] Protein-derived substances are popular conditioners for damaged hair since they can temporarily mend split ends, also medically known as trichoptilosis. Split ends arise when the protective cuticle has been lost from the distal hair shaft and the exposed cortex splits. Protein is attracted to the keratin, a property known as substantivity, and the protein adheres the cortex fragments together until the next shampooing occurs.[14]

pH adjusters

In addition to containing conditioning agents, hair shampoos contain pH adjusters to minimize hair damage from alkalinization.

Most shampoo detergents have an alkaline pH, which causes hair shaft swelling. This swelling loosens the protective cuticle, predisposing the hair shaft to damage (Figure 2.3). Hair shaft swelling can be prevented by 'pH balancing' the shampoo through the addition of an acidic substance, such as glycolic acid. Shampoos formulated at a neutral pH are most important for chemically treated hair from either permanent dyeing or permanent waving.

Specialty additives

The last and most important category of hair shampoo ingredients comprises the specialty ingredients. These additives allow the distinction of one shampoo from another in terms of marketing claims. The extra ingredients may provide unique functional attributes to the shampoo or may simply be added as the ingredient of the moment. A good example was the addition of beer during the 1970s to shampoos as a conditioner. Presently, no beer-containing shampoos are found in the mainstream market. During the 1990s manufacturers were touting the addition of glycolic acid to shampoo, even though the hair does not require exfoliation. As mentioned previously, the glycolic acid served functionally as a pH adjuster and nothing more. The current trend appears to be the addition of conditioning vitamins to shampoos, such as vitamin B5 (panthenol). Other botanicals, such as tea tree oil, have also captured the interest of the moment. It is worth mentioning that shampoos are frequently reformulated to meet the marketing expectations of the consumer.

Shampoo formulations

There are many types of shampoo, each claiming to offer the consumer a unique benefit. The basic shampoo categories are listed in Box 2.3. Shampoos have been formulated as liquids, gels, creams, aerosols, and powders; however, only the liquid formulations are discussed, since these are the most popular. Each category is discussed in detail from the perspective of the detergent classes previously presented.

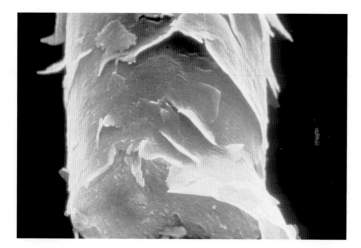

Figure 2.3
Loss of the cuticle accompanied by swelling of the cuticle through exposure of the hair to an alkaline pH result in hair shaft damage.

> **Box 2.3 Basic shampoo categories**
> - Normal hair shampoo
> - Dry hair shampoo
> - Damaged hair shampoo
> - Oily hair shampoo
> - Everyday shampoo
> - Deep cleaning shampoo
> - Baby shampoo
> - Medicated shampoo
> - Conditioning shampoo
> - Hair dyeing shampoo
> - Ethnic shampoo

Normal hair shampoo

Normal hair shampoos are designed to thoroughly cleanse the scalp and hair in persons with virgin hair and moderate sebum production. Men mainly fall into this category, although the fastest growing segment of hair dye sales is among young men! Normal hair shampoos use lauryl sulfate as the primary detergent, providing good sebum removal and minimal conditioning.

Dry hair shampoo

Dry hair shampoos provide mild cleansing and good conditioning. Some companies recommend the same product for dry hair and damaged hair. These products are excellent for mature persons and those who wish to shampoo daily. They reduce static electricity and increase manageability in fine hair; however, some products provide too much conditioning, which may result in limp hair. Dry hair shampoos may also cleanse so poorly that conditioner can build up on the hair shaft. This condition has been labeled as the 'greasies' in popular advertising and may account for the observation that hair sometimes has more body after using a different shampoo.

Damaged hair shampoo

Damaged hair shampoos are intended for hair that has been chemically treated with permanent hair colors, hair bleaching agents, permanent waving solutions or hair straighteners. Hair can also be damaged physically by overcleansing, excessive use of heated styling devices and vigorous brushing or combing. Longer hair is more likely to be damaged than shorter hair since it undergoes a natural process known as 'weathering', whereby the cuticular scales are decreased in number from the proximal to distal hair shaft (Figure 2.4). As mentioned previously, damaged hair shampoos may be identical to dry hair shampoos or may contain mild detergents and increased conditioners. Hydrolyzed animal protein is the superior conditioner for damaged hair since it can minimally penetrate the shaft and temporarily plug surface defects, resulting in hair with a smoother feel and more shine. The protein can also temporarily

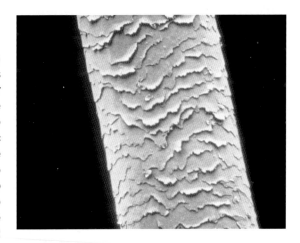

Figure 2.4
A weathered hair shaft.

mend split ends (Figure 2.5). It is important that the protein is hydrolyzed, as larger protein molecules cannot penetrate the hair shaft.

Oily hair shampoo

Oily hair shampoos have excellent cleansing and minimal conditioning properties. They may use lauryl sulfate or sulfosuccinate detergents and are intended for adolescents with oily hair or persons who have extremely dirty hair. They can be drying to the hair shaft if used daily. Following an oily hair shampoo with use of a heavy conditioner is self-defeating.

Everyday shampoo

Everyday shampoos are designed with minimal cleansing properties, since they are intended for everyday or frequent use. They are similar in formulation to dry hair shampoos, with minimal detergency and conditioning.

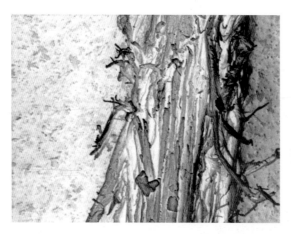

Figure 2.5
An electron micrograph of a split end.

Deep cleaning shampoo

Deep cleaning shampoos are similar to oily hair shampoos in that they are formulated with surfactants selected for their excellent sebum removal qualities. These shampoos contain no conditioning agents and are designed to be used once weekly by persons who use large amounts of hairspray, styling gels, and hair waxes for grooming (see Chapter 3).

Baby shampoo

Baby shampoos are nonirritating to the eyes and are designed as mild cleansing agents, since babies produce limited sebum. As mentioned previously, these shampoos use detergents from the amphoteric group and actually anesthetize the eye tissues, preventing stinging.[15] They are not intended for eye installation. Baby shampoos are appropriate for mature hair and for individuals who wish to shampoo daily. They are also excellent for cleansing the eyelashes in patients with ocular rosacea, ocular seborrheic dermatitis, or eye area infections.

Conditioning shampoo

Conditioning shampoos, also known as 2-in-1 shampoos, intend to both clean and condition with one product.[16,17] Detergents used in conditioning shampoos are generally amphoterics and anionics of the sulfosuccinate type. These products are designed for patients with chemically damaged hair or those who prefer to shampoo frequently.[18] Patients should not use a conditioning shampoo prior to permanent dyeing or permanent waving because maximum color uptake or curling may be inhibited.

Medicated shampoo

Medicated shampoos, also known as dandruff shampoos, contain additives such as coal tar, salicylic acid, sulfur, selenium sulfide, and zinc pyrithione.[19] These are all monographed ingredients, making this class of shampoo an over-the-counter drug. Federal guidelines stipulate that no shampoo may contain more than one of these active ingredients, prohibiting ingredient combinations that might be beneficial dermatologically. Medicated shampoos function to remove sebum, scalp scale, bacteria, and fungal elements from the scalp and hair. The shampoo base removes sebum while mechanical scrubbing removes the desquamating corneocytes[20] (Figure 2.6).

Tar derivatives are commonly used as anti-inflammatory agents. Salicylic acid is used as a keratolytic to chemically remove scalp scale. Sulfur, selenium sulfide, and zinc pyrithione are used for their antibacterial/antifungal qualities. Each of these functions is important in the prevention of seborrheic dermatitis. It is generally believed that seborrheic dermatitis is due to the overgrowth of the fungus *Malazezzia furfur*, which consumes the scalp sebum, releasing inflammatory free fatty acids as a metabolic waste product. The inflammatory free fatty acids induce scalp skin hyperproliferation and increased scale. It is for this reason that patients sometimes find benefit from rotating shampoos, each addressing a different aspect of the scalp disease.

Hair dyeing shampoo

There are special shampoos designed for use after permanent hair dyeing. These shampoos employ cationic surfactants and are formulated at an acidic pH. They are designed to neutralize any residual alkalinity from the chemicals used for hair dyeing. Bringing the hair shaft back to a neutral pH is important to decrease swelling of the hair cuticle, which should be tightly adherent to the cortex for optimum hair functioning and appearance.

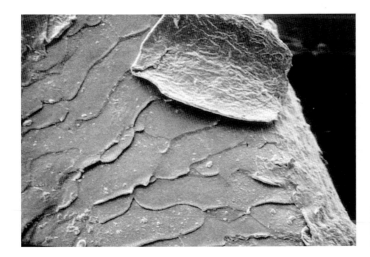

Figure 2.6
Scalp scale attached to a hair shaft seen under electron microscopy.

Ethnic shampoo

There are shampoo products specifically designed for the Black patient. These shampoos are known as conditioning shampoos, since they are formulated with both cleaning and conditioning agents, such as wheat-germ oil, steartrimonium hydrolyzed animal protein, or lanolin derivatives. They remove sebum from the hair shaft and replace it with a layer of oily conditioner to decrease combing friction of the kinky hair shafts.[21] The conditioner also increases manageability and adds shine. These shampoos are typically used once weekly or once every 2 weeks.

Shampoo-induced allergic contact dermatitis

Adverse reactions to shampoos are rare, since the product is rinsed away from the skin quickly, allowing insufficient time for the development of allergic contact dermatitis. The possible causes of allergic contact dermatitis are listed in Box 2.4.[22] Shampoo-induced allergic contact dermatitis can be confirmed by patch testing. If patch testing is required, the shampoo should be diluted to form a 1–2% aqueous solution for closed patch testing and a 5% aqueous solution for open patch testing. It is important to keep in mind that false positive reactions due to irritation may occur. A better assessment of

---

Box 2.4 Causes of shampoo-induced allergic contact dermatitis

- Formalin
- Parabens
- Hexachlorophene
- Miranols

---

shampoo-induced allergic contact dermatitis may be obtained by patch testing individual ingredients separately.[23]

CONDITIONERS

The need for hair conditioners arose following technological developments in detergents and shampoo formulation. Originally, bar soaps were used to clean both the hair and the body. Most bar soaps possessed an alkaline pH, which caused the hair shaft to swell, leaving it unattractive and unmanageable. In addition, most homes used well water for cleansing, which had a high mineral content. The combination of the bar soap and hard water yielded soap scum that accumulated on the tub and also on the hair. This soap scum left the hair harsh and dull, adding an additional source of scalp irritation.

The widespread introduction of municipal water sources and the development of liquid synthetic detergents that were formulated at a neutral pH with sequestering agents revolutionized hair shampooing. Now the shampoos left the hair soft and manageable and could be used more frequently without an adverse cosmetic result. This led to the current practice of shampooing daily or every other day, which efficiently removes sebum from the hair shaft.[24] Sebum is, of course, the ideal hair conditioner. Excessive removal of sebum created the need for a synthetic sebum-like substance able to minimize static electricity, increase hair shine, improve hair manageability, and also aid in maintaining a hairstyle. Thus, hair conditioners were developed in an attempt to supply hair with the positive attributes of sebum while avoiding the greasy appearance indicative of excessive sebum and dirty hair.

Conditioners are liquids, creams, pastes, or gels that mimic sebum in making the hair manageable, glossy, and soft. The role of conditioners goes beyond maintaining the appearance of healthy hair. Conditioners also attempt to recondition hair that has been damaged by chemical or mechanical trauma.[25] Common sources of trauma include excessive brushing, hot blow-drying, permanent hair waves, hair straightening, hair bleaching, etc. Damage to the hair shaft can also occur through environmental factors such as exposure to sunlight, air pollution, wind, seawater, and chlorinated swimming pool water.[26] This type of hair damage is technically known as 'weathering.'[27] Obviously, since hair is nonliving tissue, any reconditioning that occurs is minimal and temporary until the next shampooing.

Hair conditioners were developed during the early 1930s when self-emulsifying waxes became available. These waxes were combined with protein hydrolysates, polyunsaturates, and silicones to give the hair improved feel and texture. Early sources of protein included gelatin, milk, and egg protein.[28] Currently, the most common ingredient in hair conditioners is silicone. Silicone is a lightweight oil that can leave a thin film on the hair shaft without creating the appearance of dirty hair. The amount of silicone left behind on the hair shaft determines whether the product is designed for adding body to fine hair where minimal conditioning is desirable or straightening curly hair where maximal conditioning is desirable.

Mechanism of action

Healthy, undamaged hair is soft, resilient, and easy to disentangle.[29] Unfortunately, the trauma caused by shampooing, drying, combing, brushing, styling, dyeing, and permanent waving damages the hair, making it harsh, brittle, and difficult to disentangle.[30]

Hair conditioners are designed to reverse this hair damage by decreasing static electricity, improving manageability, increasing hair shine, decreasing split ends, and improving hair flexibility.[31] Each of these effects will be examined in detail.

Decreased static electricity

Hair conditioners improve manageability by decreasing static electricity. Following combing or brushing, the hair shafts become negatively charged. These negatively charged shafts repel one another, preventing the hair from lying smoothly in a given style. Conditioners deposit positively charged ions on the hair shaft, neutralizing the electrical charge and minimizing frizzy hair. Frizzy hair due to static electricity is a greater problem in low humidity climates, such as the southwestern United States.

Improved manageability

In addition to decreasing static electricity, hair conditioners also improve hair manageability. Manageability refers to the ease with which the hair is combed and styled. Conditioners improve manageability by decreasing the friction between hair shafts by smoothing the surface of the cuticle. This is accomplished by filling in the gaps around and between the cuticular scales. A quality hair conditioner can reduce friction between hair shafts by as much as 50%.[32] This reduction in friction also aids disentangling of the hair following shampooing leading to a subset of conditioners, known as cream rinses, designed to make hair easier to comb following shampooing. A special subset of these products is designed to aid in combing children's hair.

Increased hair shine

Most consumers equate shiny hair with healthy hair.[33] Hair shine results from light reflected by individual hair shafts.[34–36] The smoother the hair surface, the more light reflected.[37] Conditioners increase hair gloss primarily by increasing adherence of the cuticular scale to the hair shaft and placing a thin coating over the individual hairs.[38]

Decreased split ends

Conditioners can also improve the health of the hair by temporarily repairing damage at the distal hair shaft, a condition known as split ends. Split ends occur when the cuticle has been removed from the hair shaft and the soft keratin cortex and medulla are exposed to weathering and grooming trauma. The protein of these structures, unable to withstand the damage, splits or frays much like a damaged textile fiber.[39] Conditioners temporarily reapproximate the frayed remnants of remaining medulla and cortex. This strengthens the hair shaft and prevents breakage of the distal ends. However, the conditioner is removed with subsequent shampooing and must be reapplied after each shampoo contact.

Improved flexibility

Lastly, conditioners can improve hair flexibility. This is the ability of the hair to withstand the forces of bending without fracturing.[40,41] Figure 2.7 demonstrates how a hair coated with conditioner does not exhibit cuticle lifting (Figure 2.7a), while a hair devoid of conditioner shows disruption of the cuticle (Figure 2.7b). Flexibility is especially important in women with long hair to prevent hair breakage.[42]

Hair type

Even though all types of hair benefit from the use of a conditioner, conditioners must be formulated for specific hair types to function optimally.[43] There are conditioners designed for straight hair, fine hair, wavy hair, and kinky hair. It is the geometry of the hair shaft that determines the type of conditioner required to produce the best cosmetic result. For example, persons with kinky hair prefer a heavy conditioner that thickly coats the hair shaft to provide additional weight and straighten the unruly shafts. Kinky hair conditioners allow the hair to lay in the desired style while appearing shiny and healthy, but this same type of conditioner applied to fine, thin hair would make it appear greasy and limp. Fine, straight hair is best minimally conditioned, since additional straightening of the hair shafts is not a goal.

It may seem that the best way to avoid limp hair in persons with fine hair is to avoid use of a conditioner, but this is not the case. Fine hair is particularly prone to weathering and hair grooming damage. This is due to the increased number of hair fibers per weight making the net surface area of fine hair greater. This allows for proportionally more cuticular scales that can become damaged and more hair surface area that is subject to static electricity.

Formulation

The prior discussion focused on the effect of conditioners on the hair shaft, but we shall now turn to the ingredients responsible for achieving these effects.[44] There are several different active agents that can be combined to achieve a hair conditioner designed for a given hair type. The primary classes of hair conditioning agents are listed in Box 2.5.[45] Of these categories, the quaternaries,

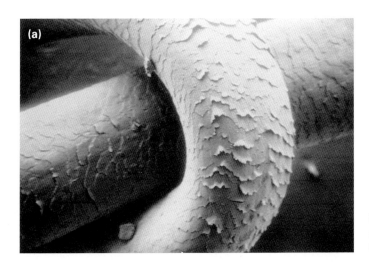

Figure 2.7
(a) A hair coated with conditioner does not exhibit cuticle lifting.

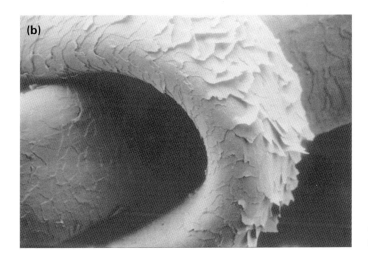

(b) A hair devoid of conditioner shows disruption of the cuticle.

polymers, and protein derivatives are the most frequently used. These more common conditioning agents are presented in Table 2.3 and are the next topic of discussion.[46]

Quaternary conditioning agents

The quaternary conditioning agents, also known as quaternaries or quaternary ammo-nium compounds or quats, are cationic detergents as discussed previously under hair shampoo detergents.[47] These ingredients are found in both conditioning shampoos and hair conditioners.[48] They function to neutralize the negative charge found on the hair shafts. Remember that hair that is susceptible to the effects of static electricity has an anionic negative charge while the quaternary conditioning agents possess a positive cationic charge.[49] The addition of the cationic quaternary conditioner neutralizes the anionic charge of the hair, decreasing static electricity and improving manageability. It is the attraction of the positively charged conditioner to the negatively charged hair shaft that allows the hair care product to remain on the hair following water rinsing.[50]

Quaternary conditioning agents are used in conditioning shampoos, also known as 2-in-1 shampoos, which clean the hair but also leave behind a thin film of conditioner to improve hair appearance. With repeated grooming and shampooing, the hair

---

Box 2.5 Hair conditioner ingredient categories

- Alkanolamides
- Glycols
- Lipids
- Quaternaries
- Polymers
- Protein derivatives
- Silicones

Table 2.3 Common hair conditioners

Hair conditioner category	Primary ingredient	Main advantage	Hair grooming benefit
Cationic detergent	Quaternary ammonium compounds	Smooth cuticle, decrease static electricity	Excellent for restoring damaged, chemically processed hair
Film-former	Polymers	Fill hair shaft defects, decrease static electricity, improve shine	Improve the appearance of dry hair, improve grooming of coarse, kinky hair
Protein-containing	Hydrolyzed proteins	Penetrate hair shaft to minimally increase strength	Temporarily mend split ends
Silicones	Dimethicone, cyclomethicone, amodimethicone	Thin coating placed on hair shafts	Decrease static electricity, decrease combing friction, add shine

becomes weathered and the cuticular scale loosened. The same effect is seen in woven textiles, such as cotton or wool sweaters, where fuzz balls and pilling occur around areas of high fabric friction, such as the elbows. These fuzz balls occur because the textile fibers have broken and rolled into a ball. The cuticular scales also fracture, break, and clump. This creates increased combing friction and hair that appears dull. Quaternary conditioners are excellent at increasing adherence of the cuticular scales to the hair shaft, which increases the light reflective abilities of the hair, adding shine and luster. These qualities make them an excellent conditioner choice for patients with permanently dyed or permanently waved hair, where the cuticle has been disrupted as part of the chemical process.

Film-forming conditioning agents

The second category of conditioning agents is known as film-formers. Rather than functioning through electrical charge, as is the case with the quaternaries, these conditioners actually coat the hair shaft with a thin layer of polymer. They contain some of the new lightweight polymers used in hairsprays and styling products, discussed in more detail in Chapter 3.[51] The most common polymer selected is polyvinylpyrrolidone, also known as PVP. The polymer forms a coating over the hair shaft to fill in hair shaft defects and missing areas of cuticular scale to create a smooth surface.[52] This smooth surface reflects increased light, thus improving hair luster and shine. In addition, the polymer coating eliminates static electricity, due to its cationic nature, also improving hair manageability.

Many of the film-forming conditioners claim to thicken hair. While consumers may think this means that more hair is present on the scalp, in actuality this claim is substantiated by measuring the diameter of each hair shaft after it has been coated by the polymer film. Indeed the hair shafts have been thickened, but not in the manner the consumer had hoped!

Film-formers are ideal in conditioners designed to straighten kinky or curly hair, since a thick coating can be applied to help straighten the hair shafts. They are also found in products to add manageability to coarse hair; however, persons with fine hair will find that the polymer coating makes the hair shaft limp and difficult to style. Film-forming conditioners are most commonly employed to hair that has been shampooed and towel-dried. They are designed to remain on the hair shaft, while the previously discussed quaternary conditioners are applied following shampooing and rinsed prior to towel-drying the hair.

Protein conditioning agents

Protein-containing conditioners are the most interesting and beneficial from a dermatologic standpoint.[53] As hair weathers, it loses its strength due to removal of the cuticular scales and damage to the underlying cortex. This damage creates areas where the hair shaft contains holes. These holes create sites for deposition of protein from a conditioner. Protein-containing conditioners can actually penetrate the damaged hair shaft and increase its fracture strength by 10%. While a 10% improvement may seem insignificant, it may make the difference between an intact hair shaft and one that is broken with the force of combing. These proteins, derived from animal collagen, keratin, placenta, etc., are hydrolyzed to a particle size of molecular weight 1000 to 10,000 Daltons, which are able to enter the hair shaft.[54] The source of the protein is not as important as the size of the protein particle and its ability to enter and remain inside the hair shaft.[55,56]

The ability of protein-containing conditioners to strengthen the hair shaft depends on contact time. The longer the protein conditioner is left in contact with the hair shaft, the more protein that will diffuse into the shaft. Thus, proteins are used in short contact instant conditioners applied after shampooing and rinsed for minimal protein penetration and in leave-on conditioners applied prior to shampooing and left on the hair for 30 minutes prior to removal for greater protein penetration. The amount of protein that penetrates the hair shaft determines the final result. However, the protein diffusion is reversible, meaning that any exogenous protein present in the hair shaft will be removed at the time of the next shampooing, necessitating reapplication of the protein-containing conditioner. Reapplication is necessary with each water contact to maintain the effect.

Silicones

The last major category of conditioning agents is silicone. Silicones have virtually revolutionized hair conditioning, both from the standpoint of conditioning shampoos and instant hair conditioners.[57] Topical silicone is an amazingly safe material from a dermatologic perspective, since it is hypoallergenic, noncomedogenic, and nonacnegenic.

Silicone was developed in the 1930s when Franklin, Hyde, and McGragor discovered a method of extracting pure silica from raw quartzite and converting it to dimethyl silicone. Silicone originates from silica, which is found in sand, quartz, and granite. It derives its properties from the alternating silica and oxygen bonds, known as siloxane bonds, which are exceedingly strong.[58]

These strong bonds account for the tremendous thermal and oxidizing stability of silicone. Silicone is resistant to decomposition from ultraviolet radiation, acids, alkalis, ozone, and electrical discharges. The silicone used in topical preparations is an odorless, colorless, nontoxic liquid. It is soluble in aromatic and halocarbon solvents, but poorly soluble in polar and aliphatic solutes. Because silicone is immiscible and insoluble in water, it is used in hair conditioners. To date there has been no report of toxicity from the use of topical silicone.

Silicone is the newest ingredient used in hair conditioners. Since silicone is water-resistant, some silicone remains on the hair shaft after water rinsing to improve manageability by reducing static electricity, minimize tangles by decreasing friction, and impart shine by smoothing roughened cuticular scale.[59-61] Since silicone can form a thin, nongreasy film on the hair shaft, it does not create the limp appearance characteristic of other hair conditioning ingredients.

Types of conditioning products

Hair conditioners are available in several types depending on their intended function and when in the grooming process they are applied.[31,62,63] The major types of hair conditioners are summarized in Table 2.4. They consist of instant conditioners, deep conditioners, leave-in conditioners, and hair rinses, the next topic of discussion.

Instant conditioners

Instant conditioners are aptly named, since they are applied directly from the bottle to the hair once it has been shampooed and rinsed. They are left in contact with the hair briefly for 1–5 minutes and then thoroughly

Table 2.4 Hair conditioner product type

Type	Use	Indication
Instant	Apply following shampoo, rinse	Minimally damaged hair, aids wet combing
Deep	Apply for 20–30 minutes, shampoo, rinse	Chemically damaged hair
Leave-in	Apply to towel-dried hair, style	Prevent hairdryer damage, aid in combing and styling
Rinse	Apply following shampoo, rinse	Aid in disentangling if creamy rinse, remove soap residue if clear rinse

rinsed. Due to their short contact time, they provide minimal conditioning and must be used after each shampooing to achieve the desired effect. The need for instant hair conditioners arose after hair shampoo detergents were developed with excellent sebum-removing capabilities. In addition, many of the currently popular hair styles require frequent shampooing to remove the styling gels, mousses, waxes, and sprays. Thus, the hair must be shampooed daily with a strong detergent, which leaves the hair unmanageable. Instant conditioners are used by persons who shampoo frequently and who have hair damaged by permanent waving or dyeing chemical processes.

Instant conditioners are the most popular type of hair conditioner for both home and salon use, even though they have limited ability to repair damaged hair. They contain water, conditioning agents, lipids, and thickeners. The conditioning agent usually consists of cationic detergent, known as quats, discussed previously.

Deep conditioners

Deep conditioners are generally creams or oils, in contrast to instant conditioners which are generally lotions, and are designed to remain on the hair for 20–30 minutes prior to shampoo removal. They usually contain higher concentrations of the quaternary and protein-containing conditioning agents.[64] Deep conditioners for African-American individuals with kinky hair may consist of warm oil applied to the hair shaft (Figure 2.8). The goal of a deep conditioner is to allow the conditioning agent to more thoroughly coat and penetrate the hair shaft to improve its cosmetic appearance.[65]

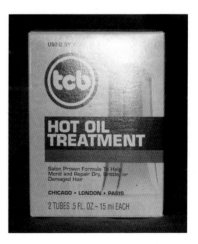

Figure 2.8
A hot oil treatment for the conditioning of kinky hair.

Sometimes heat is used to enhance penetration in the form of a hairdryer or warm towel to cause hair shaft swelling, which allows increased conditioner penetration.

These products are intended for extremely dry and damaged hair. Many patients who present to the dermatologist complaining of hair loss are actually experiencing hair breakage and not true hair loss from the follicle. These patients have subjected their hair to too much manipulation, both chemical and physical, for the hair fiber to maintain its strength. Specialized deep conditioners, known as fillers, can be recommended to these patients to minimize the hair damage from additional chemical processing. Fillers are designed to condition the distal hair shaft and reverse some of the effects of hair damage, allowing even application of the subsequent coloring or waving procedure.

Leave-in conditioners

Leave-in conditioners are applied following towel-drying of the hair and are designed to remain on the hair shaft to aid in styling. They are removed with the next shampooing. A large category of leave-in conditioners, known as blow-drying lotions, are designed to coat the hair shaft and protect the hair protein from heat damage during the drying process.

The most popular leave-in hair conditioners are designed for persons with curly or kinky hair. These products lubricate and moisturize the hair shaft while aiding in styling. For example, oil sheen sprays and oily pomades help retain water within chemically straightened hair shafts and decrease the combing friction between hair shafts, thereby preventing hair breakage. For persons with fine, straight hair, the oily leave-in conditioner would render the hair limp and hard to style, but for persons with coarse kinky hair, the oils improve manageability and impart shine. These products typically contain petrolatum, mineral oil, vegetable oils, and silicone, and function as a true hair moisturizer.

Hair rinses

Hair rinses are a special category of hair conditioners designed as thin liquids applied like an instant hair conditioner after shampooing and rinsed. They utilize cationic quaternary ammonium compounds, such as stearalkonium chloride and benzalkonium chloride. These products mainly facilitate hair detangling by reducing friction and do little else to condition the hair shaft. They are intended for persons with oily hair who need little conditioning due to abundant sebum production.

Conditioners and photoprotection

Some conditioners incorporate sunscreens to provide hair photoprotection.[66,67] This is a rather controversial subject, since the hair is nonliving and cannot undergo carcinogenesis. Hair photoprotection is basically to preserve the cosmetic value of the hair as a textile fiber.[68,69] Hair dryness, reduced strength, rough surface texture, loss of color, decreased luster, stiffness, and brittleness are all precipitated by sun exposure.[70]

Hair protein degradation is induced by light wavelengths from 254 to 400 nm.[71,72] Chemically, these changes are thought to be due to ultraviolet light-induced oxidation of the sulfur molecules within the hair shaft.[73,74] Oxidation of the amide carbon of polypeptide chains also occurs, producing carbonyl groups in the hair shaft.[75] This process has been studied extensively in wool fibers where it is known as 'photoyellowing.'[76,77]

Bleaching, or lightening of the hair color, is common in individuals who expose their hair to ultraviolet radiation.[78,79] Brunette hair tends to develop reddish hues due to photo-oxidation of melanin pigments, while blond hair develops undesirable yellow tones.[80] The yellow discoloration is due to photodegradation of cystine, tyrosine, and tryptophan residues within the blond hair shaft.[81] In addition, hair treated with permanent or semipermanent hair dyes may also shift color when exposed to sunlight.[82–85]

Sunscreen-containing conditioners are available; however, there is some debate as to their effectiveness in protecting the hair and the scalp.[86] In order to develop a standardized rating system for hair products, the concept of HPF, or hair protection factor, has been proposed.[87] This is similar to the concept of SPF, or skin protection factor, except that tensile strength assessments of the hair shaft are used for grading instead of sunburn assessment. HPF ratings follow a logarithmic scale from 2 to 15. At present, shampoo formulations containing octyldimethyl PABA and hairspray formulations containing benzophenones have been proposed.[88] Both of these products seem to decrease ultraviolet light-induced melanin and keratin damage, thus preserving the color and structure of the hair shaft.[88] At present, however, hair conditioners do not typically contain sunscreens due to the sticky feel they impart to the clean hair shafts.

Contact dermatitis

The last issue to consider is contact dermatitis associated with hair conditioners. The incidence is remarkably small. This is due to the fact that hair conditioners are applied to the hair and rinsed quickly, allowing minimal time for any reaction to occur. Rarely, hair conditioners can cause eye and skin irritation.[89] If patch testing is required, these products can be patch tested 'as is' in an open or closed manner.

HAIR DRYING

We have discussed methods of cleansing and conditioning the hair. Our attention now turns to methods of drying the hair. Hair drying is actually a fairly complex physical reaction, since the hair contains abundant water reformable bonds. These bonds reform as the hair dries in the configuration of the hair shaft the instant before drying. This means that drying is not only a technique for removing water from the hair shafts, but also a method of hair styling.

The devices used for hair drying are the hand-held hairdryer (Figure 2.9) and the hood hairdryer (Figure 2.10). The hand-held hairdryer usually comes with three heat settings: cold, warm, and hot. Since the hair is made up of protein, it is possible to denature it with excessive heat. Thus, the hairdryer should be used on warm to prevent hair heat damage. While this slows down the drying process, it will prevent unnecessary hair damage. Figure 2.11 demonstrates the steps for hair drying with a hand-held dryer. Holding the hand-held dryer too close to the hair shafts also results in hair damage (Figures 2.12 and 2.13).

The hairdryer can also be used as a styling device. The fingers can be used with a hairdryer to produce a final hairstyle. Round brushes can be used to curl the hair during the drying process (Figures 2.14 and 2.15) or the hair can be pulled straight, if desired.

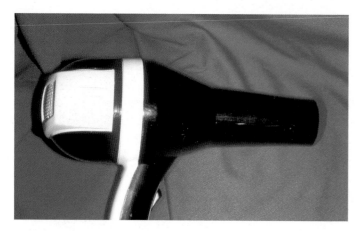

Figure 2.9
Hand-held hairdryer.

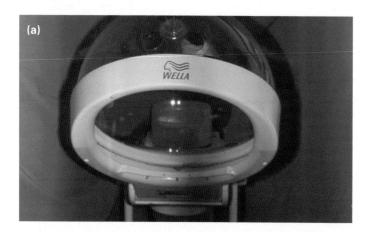

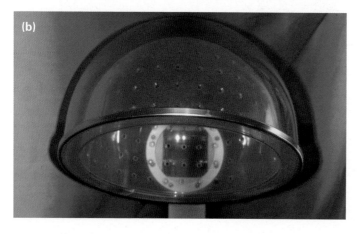

Figure 2.10
(a and b) Two different types of salon
hood hairdryers.

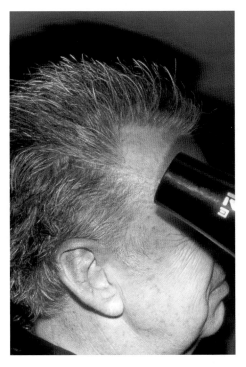

Figure 2.11
Hand-held hairdryer technique.

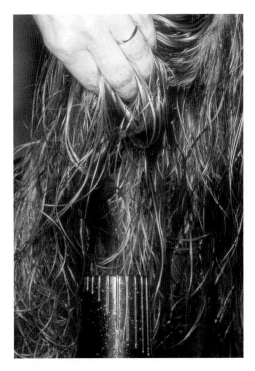

Figure 2.12
Handryer close to hair.

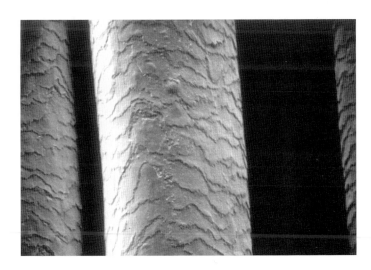

Figure 2.13
An electron micrograph demonstrating small bubbles that have developed in a wavy hair shaft from excessive hairdryer heat.

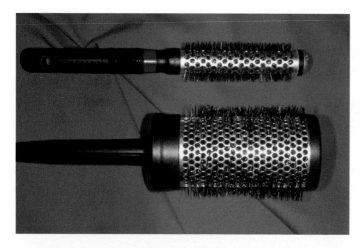

Figure 2.14
An example of a round brush used to dry hair.

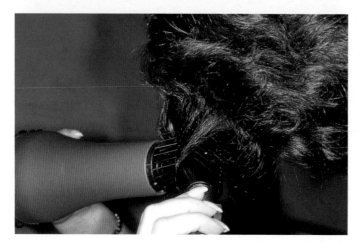

Figure 2.15
Round brush-aided hairdrying.

COMBING AND BRUSHING

Combing and brushing are activities that can either occur concurrently with hair drying, as part of the styling process following hair drying, or for grooming purposes in between hair cleansing. There are a tremendous variety of combs and brushes on the market, each designed with a specific purpose in mind (Figure 2.16). This section will look at the various grooming implements.

Combs are the most important grooming implements for detangling the hair both when wet and dry. Figure 2.17 shows a well designed comb for grooming long female hair, with a sturdy handle and widely spaced teeth. This latter comb has teeth that are too long to comb shorter male hair, but Figure 2.18 shows a better design for men. Figure 2.19 shows a relatively new comb design for detangling both male and female hair, with broadly spaced Teflon-coated teeth to minimize hair combing friction. Special hair picks have been designed for kinky African-American hair (Figure 2.20).

While some combs are designed for detangling, other combs are intended to

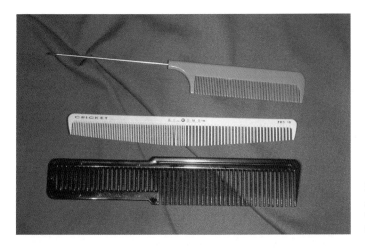

Figure 2.16
An example of the tremendous variety of hair combs presently on the market.

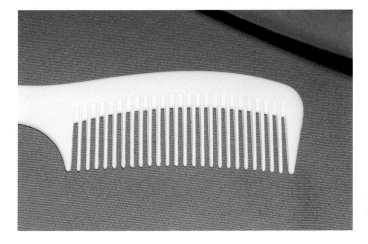

Figure 2.17
Well-designed comb for grooming long hair.

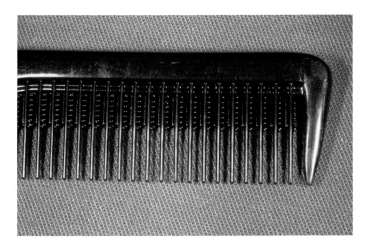

Figure 2.18
Male short hair comb.

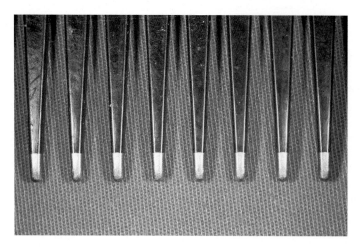

Figure 2.19
Detangling comb.

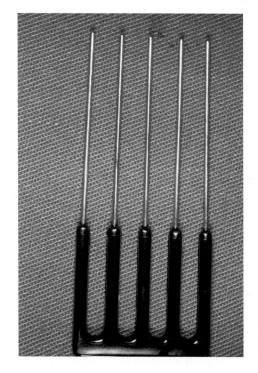

Figure 2.20
A hair pick.

create knots as part of a combing technique known as teasing (Figure 2.21). Hair is traditionally combed from the proximal to distal ends; however, in teasing the hair is combed in the opposite direction from proximal to distal. For this reason, hair teasing is also known as backcombing. Teasing is used to create the appearance of increased hair volume by creating tangles to increase the volume of the hair on the head. Teasing is particularly popular among mature women with thinning hair who have their hair shampooed and styled weekly in the salon. Figure 2.22 shows a teasing comb with closely spaced teeth of different lengths. This comb produces extensive hair damage when used because the cuticle is lifted and sometimes removed.[90] Figure 2.23 shows a teasing comb with wide-spaced Teflon-coated teeth that is less damaging, but still not recommended for hair grooming.

Brushes are also used for hair grooming. They cause more hair damage than combs owing to the closely spaced bristles that can

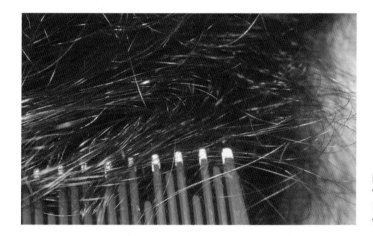

Figure 2.21
The appearance of knots intentionally created in the hair with the aid of a teasing comb.

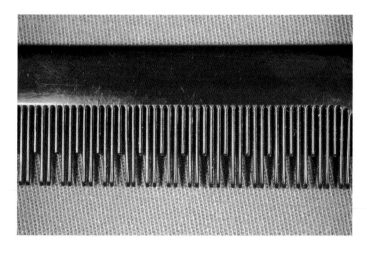

Figure 2.22
Salon teasing comb.

both fracture the hair shafts and remove the cuticle. Hairbrushes come in two types: flexible bristle and stiff bristle. Figure 2.24 shows two types of flexible bristle brushes – plastic bristles and ball-tipped bristles. Notice how the plastic bristles have pointed tips (Figure 2.25) that can tear the hair shafts. In order to reduce the chances of hair breakage, newer flexible bristle brushes with ball tips have been developed (Figure 2.26). These are the preferred brushes for grooming short and long male and female hair.

Figure 2.27 demonstrates the stiff bristle brushes. These particular brushes are round and used for curling the hair while blow-drying. Notice the holes in the brush base. These holes are designed to allow the hot air from the hairdryer to pass through the brush rather than concentrating on the brush base (Figure 2.28). This design prevents the hair from unnecessary heat damage during styling while blow-drying. In general, stiff bristle brushes are not recommended for hairstyling, since they tend to increase hair breakage (Figure 2.29).

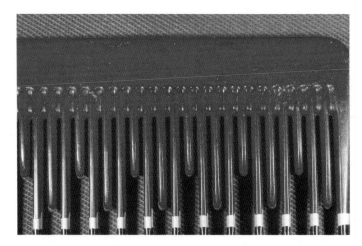

Figure 2.23
Less damaging teasing comb.

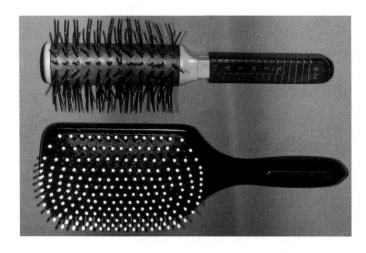

Figure 2.24
Flexible bristle brushes.

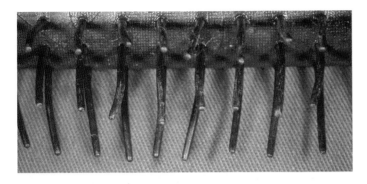

Figure 2.25
Plastic flexible bristle brush.

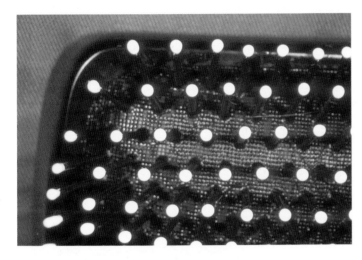

Figure 2.26
Ball-tipped flexible bristle brush.

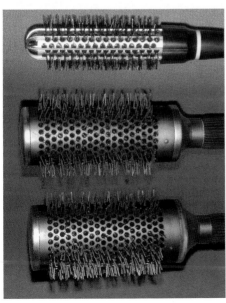

Figure 2.27
Stiff bristle brushes for blow-drying.

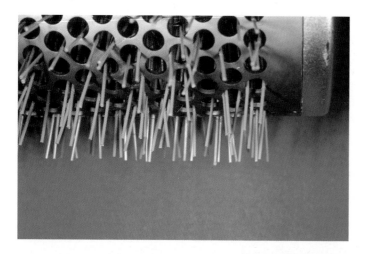

Figure 2.28
Vented round blow-drying brush.

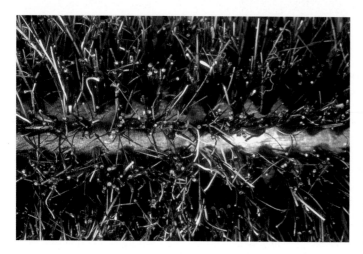

Figure 2.29
Broken hairs can be seen in this stiff bristle brush.

HAIRSTYLING

Hairstyling is one of the biggest modern preoccupations of both men and women. The major part of hairstyling would have to be the haircut, which can cost anywhere from $5 up to $500. Everyone is searching for the perfect haircut that will accentuate positive features, create the appearance of abundant hair, and compliment an overall attractive appearance. This section reviews the currently popular implements for hair cutting and pictorially discusses hair-cutting techniques for short female hair, long female hair, and male hair.

Hair-cutting implements

The main implements used to cut hair are the scissors, razor blade, and electrical clippers. Scissors come in a variety of designs, each created for a specific purpose (Figure 2.30). Basic hair-cutting scissors have a short handle and straight short blades designed to fit in the hand of the hairstylist. Sharp scissors are essential to preventing distal hair shaft damage, since dull scissors can crush the hair shaft and precipitate split ends (Figure 2.31). Specialized scissors, known as thinning shears, are used to cut and thin the hair in persons with exceptionally thick hair. Figure 2.32 demonstrates the thinning shears blade, which is notched and toothed at the tip to create numerous fine cutting edges. These multiple cutting edges prevent the scissors from binding when cutting very thick hair. Thinning shears are most commonly used when cutting the hair of preadolescent boys. The last type of scissors is a

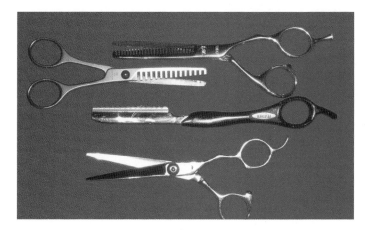

Figure 2.30
A variety of hair-cutting scissors.

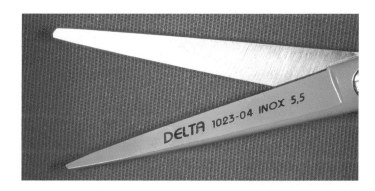

Figure 2.31
Basic hair-cutting scissors blades.

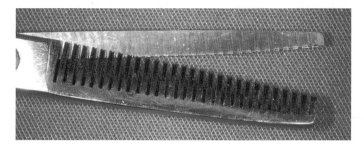

Figure 2.32
Thinning shears blades.

notched scissors as demonstrated in Figure 2.33. Notice that the blades are discontinuous. This type of scissors is designed to cut some hairs and not others. These scissors are used to create the irregular bangs (fringes) popular in children and some adolescents.

In addition to scissors, razor blades are also used to cut the hair. Some stylists feel that scissors do not cut the hair cleanly and accurately and use nothing but a hand-held straight edge for hair cutting (Figure 2.34). It is true that the razor blade produces a sharper cut (Figure 2.35), but the time to complete a razor blade cut is quite long, making these haircuts more expensive. It is unclear where they offer a true advantage to the average person with healthy hair. Razor blades are sometimes used to shave the neck and sideburns of men, where they are well suited to achieving a close cut (Figure 2.36).

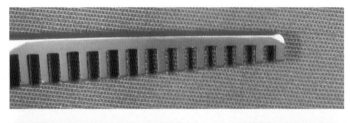

Figure 2.33
Notched scissors.

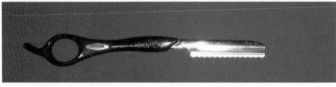

Figure 2.34
Hand-held single-edged razor blade.

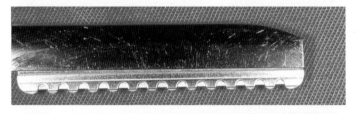

Figure 2.35
Close-up view of hair-cutting razor blade.

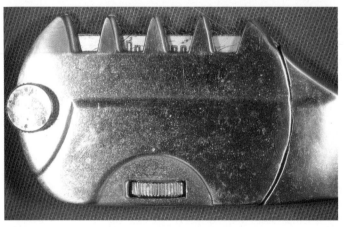

Figure 2.36
Razor blade for shaving the male neck.

Scissors and razors can be used to cut and shape the hair, but electric clippers are used to cut the hair, as well as shave the sideburns and neck of males. In Figure 2.37, the electric clippers have been fitted with a special guide designed to achieve a short male haircut where all the hairs are cut to the same length. This type of haircut is sometimes known as a 'crew-cut' or a 'buzz cut'.

Hair-cutting techniques

The art of the haircut is certainly a driving force in the salon industry. While there are many different styling methods, three different types of haircuts are presented to give the physician reader a basic idea of elements common to all haircuts. Hair-cutting techniques are described for short female hair, long female hair, and short male hair.

Short female hair is basically cut in three sections: back, sides, and bangs. The back is generally cut first in sections. It is very difficult to get all hairs of the same length on the back of the head where the hair is the thickest. For this reason, the hair is divided in sections, such as right lower, left lower, right middle, left middle, right upper, and right lower posterior head. Figure 2.38 demonstrates how the hair is sectioned and divided via the use of hair clips. This same dividing technique is used to cut the bangs and the sides of the head.

Long female hair is cut in a similar fashion, as demonstrated in Figure 2.39. The hair can be held at different angles to achieve the various lengths on different parts of the scalp which yield a final hairstyle. The hair can be held between the fingers in an angled fashion to achieve hair tapering or it can be twisted to achieve hairs of many different lengths. These techniques are basically the art of the hairstyle.

Lastly, a male haircut is demonstrated in Figure 2.40. The male haircut is actually more complex, because the hair on the head must be cut while the hair of the sideburns and neck must be shaved. The hair must also be tapered around the ears and blended into the neck and sideburns. Most male haircuts are achieved by cutting the hair the same length over the entire scalp. This creates the illusion of hair fullness and allows the hair to lie in an even organized fashion.

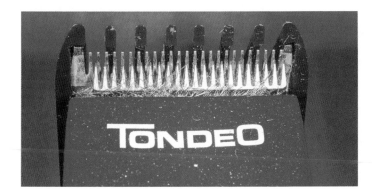

Figure 2.37
Electric clippers for cutting hair with guide.

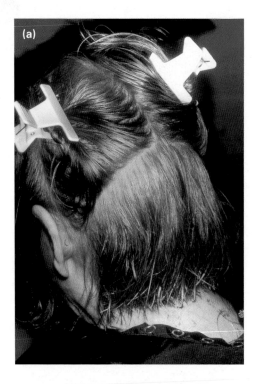

Figure 2.38
Short female haircut. (a) Hair divided on the
posterior scalp.

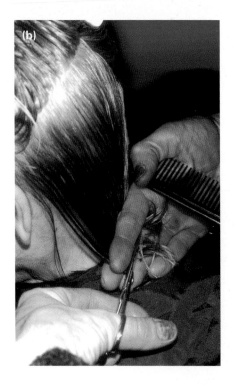

(b) Hair held tightly between first and second
fingers to obtain a straight line for cutting.

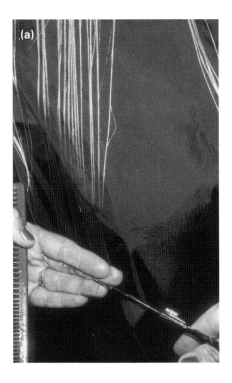

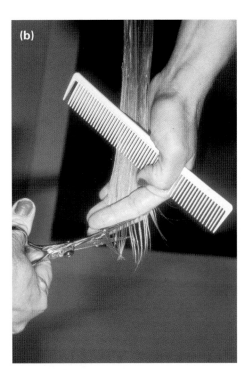

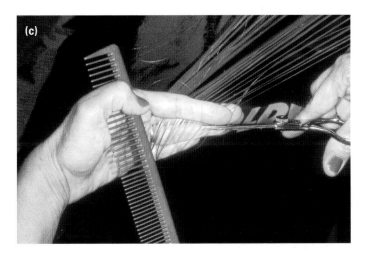

Figure 2.39
Long female haircut. (a) The back of the head is cut. (b) The sides of the head are cut. (c) Hair is angled to achieve a tapered cut.

Figure 2.39 continued

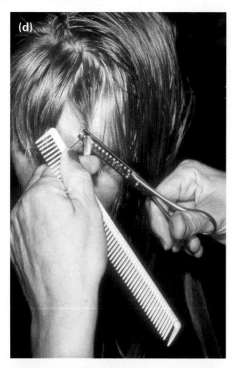

(d) Bangs are cut with hair twisted to obtain hairs of uneven length.

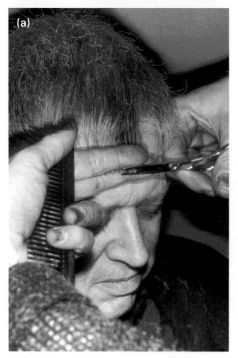

Figure 2.40
Male short haircut. (a, b, c) Hair is cut to an even length between the first and second fingers.
(d) Sideburn area is shaved with electric clippers.
(e) Neck is shaved with electric clippers.

Figure 2.40 continued

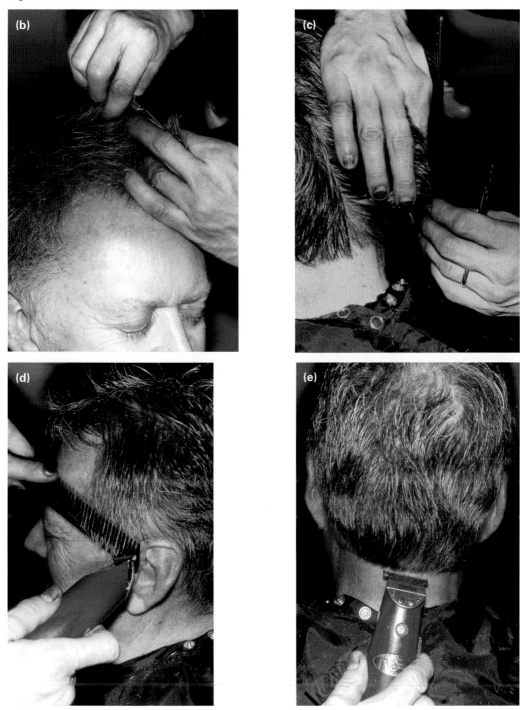

Figure 2.40 continued

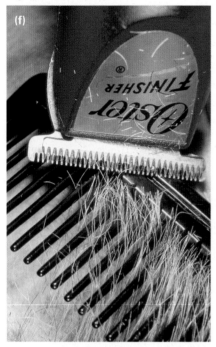

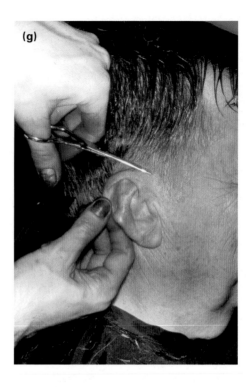

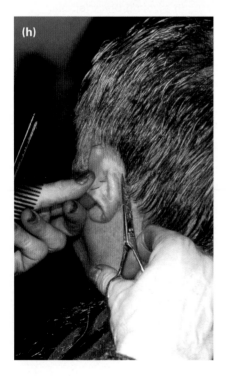

(f) Electric clippers cutting neck hair. (g) Hair is trimmed in front of the ear. (h) Hair at the back of the ear is trimmed.

Hair braiding and twisting techniques

In addition to cutting the hair to a manageable shape, hair can also be twisted or braided to obtain the desired style. Twisting and braiding are common hairstyling techniques in Black individuals with kinky hair shafts. Twisting involves sectioning the hair into quadrants on the top, sides, and posterior scalp followed by twirling of the hair into a small ponytail that is secured with a rubber band or clasp (Figure 2.41). It is important not to pull the hair too tightly or traction alopecia may result[91] (Figure 2.42).

Braiding may be performed either off or on the scalp. Braiding off the scalp is similar to the twisting technique previously described, except that the ponytail of hair is braided. Conversely, braiding on the scalp is a technique also known as 'cornrowing.' Cornrowing involves plaiting the hair by adding strands from the scalp as the braid is constructed to create a tightly adherent braid in various patterns over the scalp (Figure 2.43). Synthetic hair can also be woven into the braids, a technique discussed in the chapter on hair additions (page 174). Usually, the braids are worn for

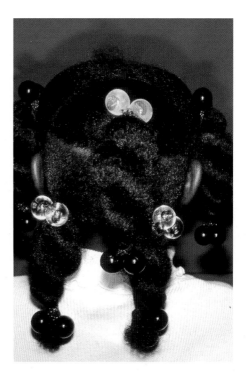

Figure 2.41
Hair twisting in a young Black female.

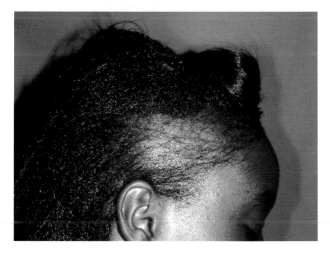

Figure 2.42
Traction alopecia may occur as a result of prolonged tight hair twisting.

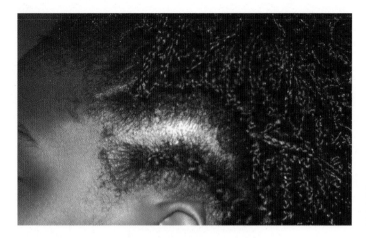

Figure 2.43
Braiding on the scalp of a young
Black female.

2–4 weeks and then undone and rebraided, if
desired (Figure 2.44). This continuous tension on the hair shaft can also result in traction alopecia, especially at the temples.[92–95]

HAIRSTYLING IMPLEMENTS AND DEVICES

Once the hair has been cut, it must be styled
to achieve the final appearance. This can be
accomplished with either nonelectric styling
implements or electric styling devices.
Nonelectric styling implements include dry
rollers, while electric styling devices include
curling irons, crimping irons, and electric
curlers.

Nonelectric styling implements

Hair curling is considered essential by most
women to achieve a fashionable hairstyle. A
curl is created by reshaping either water-
reformable bonds or heat-reformable bonds.
We shall first consider the technique used to
alter the water-reformable bonds through
the use of dry rollers.

It is first necessary to understand the
physical changes that occur when hair goes
from wet to dry under tension. Hair is made

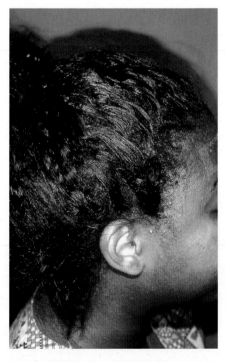

Figure 2.44
Braiding off the scalp with the
addition of synthetic hair fibers to
create volume and fullness.

up of keratin that is normally present in an alpha configuration. With tension, however, the normal alpha-keratin bond structure is changed to a beta-keratin structure. Wet hair is more elastic than dry hair, which allows partial transformation of the normal alpha-keratin structure to a beta-keratin structure when the hair is placed under tension. This transformation shifts the relative position of the polypeptide chains and brings about a disruption of ionic and hydrogen bonds. During the drying process, new ionic and hydrogen bonds are formed, blocking return to the natural alpha-keratin configuration and allowing the hair to remain in its newly curled position (Figure 2.45). Wetting the hair, however, returns hair bonds immediately to the natural alpha configuration.[96]

Hair must be rolled under tension to provide the load required for bond breakage, but the hair should not be stretched beyond the point at which more than one-third of the alpha-keratin bonds have been unfolded to beta-keratin bonds. Excessive stretching will result in permanent deformation transforming the normally elastic hair shaft into a

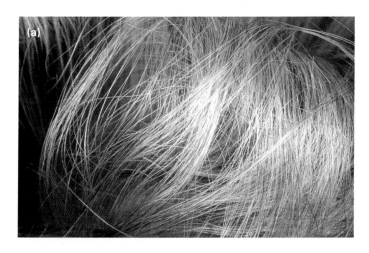

Figure 2.45
Wet hair curling process. (a) Hair straight in the alpha-keratin configuration.

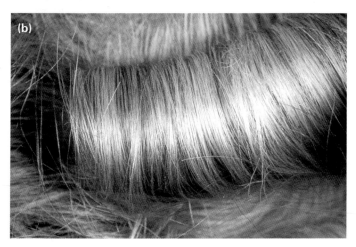

(b) Hair curled in the beta-keratin configuration.

brittle hair shaft, which will ultimately result in hair shaft fracture. The hair is typically wound around rollers, with small rollers creating small curls (Figure 2.46) and large rollers creating large curls (Figure 2.47). The rollers are placed in the desired location over the scalp to create the intended hairstyle (Figure 2.48). Rollers are available in a brush variety (Figure 2.49) and a smooth variety (Figure 2.50). Brush rollers remain in place without the use of clips required for securing the smooth rollers (Figure 2.51) and are the most popular rollers used in professional hair salons; however, they tend to cause more hair breakage as the hair gets caught in the closely spaced teeth. Smooth rollers are recommended for patients with thinning fragile hair.

Electric styling implements

In addition to water-reformable bonds, the hair also contains heat-reformable bonds, leading to the development of electric hairstyling implements. The most popular implement used for heated hairstyling is the

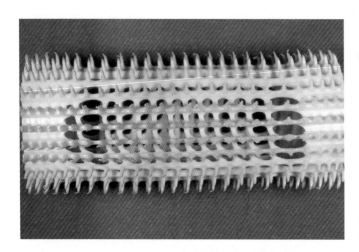

Figure 2.46
Small brush roller.

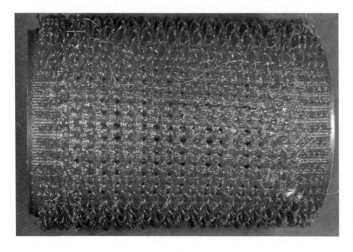

Figure 2.47
Large brush roller.

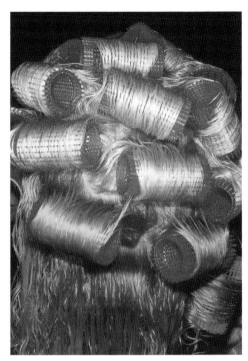

Figure 2.48
Rollers in place to curl
entire head of hair.

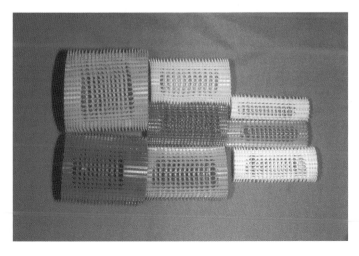

Figure 2.49
Brush rollers.

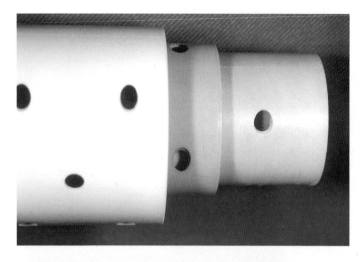

Figure 2.50
Smooth rollers.

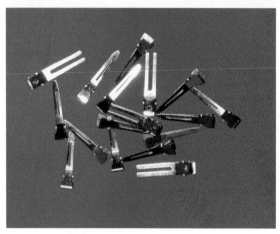

Figure 2.51
Hair clips for smooth rollers.

curling iron, which is a modern version of the oven-heated metal rods that were wrapped with hair in the pre-electric era. Modern electric curling irons are thermostatically controlled rods of varying sizes around which the hair is wrapped (Figure 2.52). Small curling rods make small curls while large curling rods make larger curls. The hair is affixed to the rod with a clip (Figure 2.53) and then wound with slight tension around the mandrel (Figure 2.54). Most curling irons produce temperatures capable of producing a deep first or superficial second degree skin burn. They are also capable

of burning the hair.[97] Some irons come with variable temperature settings, but most patients prefer the hottest setting since the curls produced are tighter and longer-lasting. It is recommended that patients remove excess heat from the curling iron prior to use by placing it in a moist towel. This lowers the rod temperature, preventing burns of the hair and scalp.

A curling iron technique used by African-American women is the Marcel iron (Figure 2.55). This is a curling iron that is used to create gentle waves in hair that has been chemically relaxed. Marceling is used in

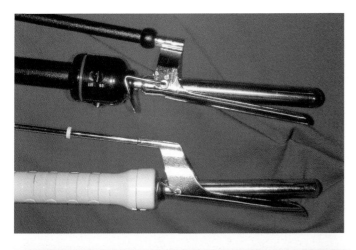

Figure 2.52
Various sized curling irons.

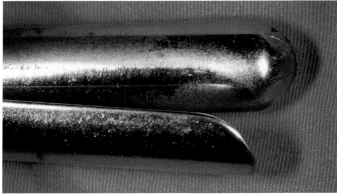

Figure 2.53
Curling rod clip.

both men and women (Figure 2.56). Recently, this hairstyling has seen a resurgence of popularity.

A variation of the curling iron is the hair iron (Figure 2.57). It consists of two heated hinged metal plates between which the hair is placed. If the plates are corrugated, the device is known as a crimping iron and produces tight bends in the hair shaft. If the plates are smooth, the device is known as a hair iron for straightening kinky hair.

Another heat-straightening device for those with kinky hair is a hot comb, developed by Madame C.J. Walker, who is credited with originating the ethnic hair care industry.[98] Hot combing employs a metal comb that is heated to a minimum of 300 degrees Fahrenheit and drawn through the hair. This breaks the heat-reformable bonds, composed of hydrogen bonds and salt linkages, allowing the hair to be pulled straight. The change is temporary, however, as moisture from perspiration, humidity or shampooing allows the bonds to reform and the hair returns to its natural kinky state.[99] Thus, heat-straightening techniques are temporary, but can be improved if a pressing oil is added to the hair prior to hot combing or ironing. The pressing oil improves water resistance and contains oily substances such as petrolatum, mineral oil, ceresin wax, or cetyl alcohol. It may also

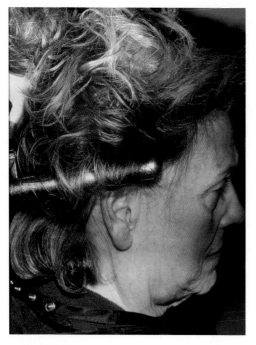

Figure 2.54
Hair wound on curling iron.

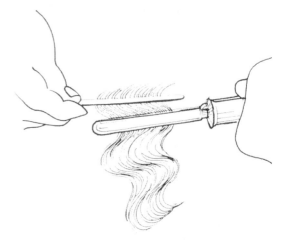

Figure 2.55
A diagram illustrating the Marcel technique.

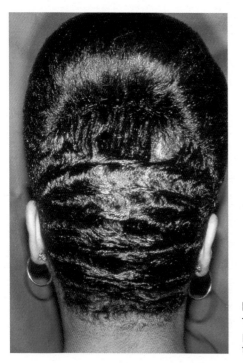

Figure 2.56
The appearance of the hair on the posterior scalp after using the Marcel technique.

contribute to hot comb alopecia;[100] however, there is some controversy as to whether all cases of scarring alopecia in Black patients who use heat straightening represent hot comb alopecia or the newly described follicular degeneration syndrome.[101] Temporary heat straightening remains popular since it is inexpensive and can be performed at home.

The last electric styling implement to be discussed is electric curlers, which are individually heated, plastic-coated rods of varying sizes (Figure 2.58). They are actually safer than a curling iron, due to the plastic coating over the metal core that prevents scalp and skin burns. Electric curlers do not produce as tight a curl, since the hair is exposed to lower temperatures. Higher heat produces tighter curls, but also more hair damage. There is a condition, known as bubble hair, discussed in Chapter 7 where heated devices, such as curlers, actually boil the water within the hair shaft causing cuticle damage. The best way to prevent heat-induced hair damage from electric curlers is to unplug the curlers for a few minutes to allow cooling prior to placing the warm curler in the hair.

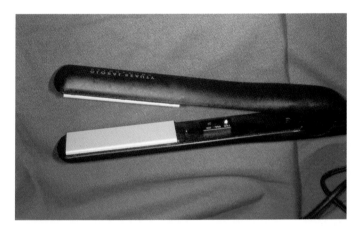

Figure 2.57
An example of a hair iron for straightening kinky hair.

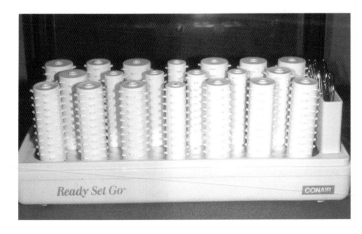

Figure 2.58
Electric heated curlers.

REFERENCES

1. Robbins CR. Interaction of shampoo and creme rinse ingredients with human hair. In: *Chemical and physical behavior of human hair*, 2nd edn. New York: Springer-Verlag, 1988;122–67.
2. Westman M. New shampoo technologies: between the shock waves. *Cosmet Toilet* 2003;**118**:58–63.
3. Bouillon C. Shampoos and hair conditioners. *Clin Dermatol* 1988;**6**:83–92.
4. Markland WR. Shampoos. In: de Navarre MG, ed. *The chemistry and manufacture of cosmetics*, Vol IV, 2nd edn. Wheaton IL: Allured Publishing Corporation, 1988;1283–312.
5. Fox C. An introduction to the formulation of shampoos. *Cosmet Toilet* 1988;**103**:25–58.
6. Zviak C, Vanlerberghe G. Scalp and hair hygiene. In: Zviak C, ed. *The science of hair care*. New York: Marcel Dekker, 1986;49–86.
7. Shipp JJ. Hair-care products. In: Williams DF, Schmitt WH, eds. *Chemistry and technology of the cosmetics and toiletries industry*. London: Blackie Academic & Professional, 1992;32–54.
8. Tokiwa F, Hayashi S, Okumura T. Hair and surfactants. In: Kobori T, Montagna W, eds. *Biology and disease of the hair*. Baltimore: University Park Press, 1975;631–40.
9. Bouillon C. Shampoos and hair conditioners. *Clin Dermatol* 1988;**6**:83–92.
10. Powers DH. Shampoos. In: Balsam MS, Gershon SD, Reiger MM, Sagarin E, Strianse SJ, eds. *Cosmetics science and technology*. 2nd edn. New York: Wiley-Interscience, 1972: 73–116.
11. Zviak C, Vanlerberghe G. Scalp and hair hygiene. In: Zviak C, ed. *The science of hair care*. New York: Marcel Dekker, 1986:49–86.
12. Harusawa F, Nakama Y, Tanaka M. Anionic-cationic ion-pairs as conditioning agents in shampoos. *Cosmet Toilet* 1991;**106**:35–39.
13. Sun J, Parr J, Travagline D. Stable conditioning shampoos containing high molecular weight dimethicone. *Cosmet Toilet* 2002; **117**:41–50.
14. Karjala SA, Williamson JE, Karler A. Studies on the substantivity of collagen-derived pep-tides to human hair. *J Soc Cosmet Chem* 1966;**17**:513–24.
15. Wilkinson JB, Moore RJ. *Harry's cosmeticology*. New York: Chemical Publishing, 1982: 457–8.
16. Hunting ALL. Can there be cleaning and conditioning in the same product? *Cosmet Toilet* 1988;**103**:73–8.
17. Gruber J, Lamoureux B, Joshi N, Moral L. The use of x-ray fluorescent spectroscopy to study the influence of cationic polymers on silicone oil deposition from shampoo. *J Cosmet Sci* 2001;**52**:131–6.
18. Lochhead R. Formulating conditioning shampoos. *Cosmet Toilet* 2001;**116**:55–66.
19. Spoor HJ. Shampoos. *Cutis* 1973;**12**:671–2.
20. Pierard-Franchimont C, Arrese J, Pierard G. Sebum flow dynamics and antidandruff shampoos. *J Soc Cosmet Chem* 1997;**48**: 117–21.
21. Brooks G, Burmeister F. Black hair care ingredients. *Cosmet Toilet* 1988;**103**:93–6.
22. Bergfeld WF. The side effects of hair products on the scalp and hair. In: Orfanos CE, Montagna W, Stuttgen G, eds. *Hair research*. New York: Springer-Verlag, 1981:507–11.
23. De Groot AC, Weyland JW, Nater JP. *Unwanted effects of cosmetics and drugs used in dermatology*. Amsterdam: Elsevier, 1994:473–6.
24. Goldemberg RL. Hair conditioners: the rationale for modern formulations. In: Frost P, Horwitz SN, eds. *Principles of cosmetics for the dermatologist*. St Louis: CV Mosby Company, 1982:157–9.
25. Swift JA, Brown AC. The critical determination of fine change in the surface architecture of human hair due to cosmetic treatment. *J Soc Cosmet Chem* 1972;**23**:675–702.
26. Zviak C, Bouillon C. Hair treatment and hair care products. In: Zviak C, ed. *The science of hair care*. New York: Marcel Dekker, 1986:115–16.
27. Rook A. The clinical importance of 'weathering' in human hair. *Br J Dermatol* 1976; **95**:111–12.
28. deNavarre MG. Hair conditioners and rinses. In: deNavarre MG, ed. *The chemistry and manufacture of cosmetics*, Vol IV, 2nd edn. Wheaton, IL: Allured Publishing 1988: 1097–109.

29. Garcia ML, Epps JA, Yare RS, Hunter LD. Normal cuticle-wear patterns in human hair. *J Soc Cosmet Chem* 1978;**29**:155–75.
30. Corbett JF. Hair conditioning. *Cutis* 1979;**23**:405–13.
31. Klein K. Formulating hair conditioners: hope and hype. *Cosmet Toilet* 2003;**118**:28–31.
32. Price VH. The role of hair care products. In: Orfanos CE, Montagna W, Stuttgen G, eds. *Hair research*. Berlin: Springer-Verlag, 1981: 501–6.
33. McMullen R, Jachowicz J. Optical properties of hair: effect of treatments on luster as quantified by image analysis. *J Cosmet Sci* 2003;**54**:335–51.
34. Okamoto M, Yakawa R, Mamada A *et al.* Influence of internal structures of hair fiber on hair appearance. III. Generation of light-scattering factors in hair cuticles and the influence on hair shine. *J Cosmet Sci* 2003;**54**:353–66.
35. Tango Y, Shimmoto K. Development of a device to measure human hair luster. *J Cosmet Sci* 2001;**52**:237–50.
36. Scanavez C, Zoega M, Barbosa A, Joekes I. Measurement of hair luster by diffuse reflectance spectrophotometry. *J Cosmet Sci* 2000;**51**:289–302.
37. Robinson VNE. A study of damaged hair. *J Soc Cosmet Chem* 1976;**27**:155–61.
38. Zviak C, Bouillon C. Hair treatment and hair care products. In: Zviak C, ed. *The science of hair care*. New York: Marcel Dekker, 1986: 134–7.
39. Swift J. Mechanism of split-end formation in human head hair. *J Soc Cosmet Chem* 1997;**48**:123–6.
40. Baltenneck F, Franbourg A, Leroy F, Mandon M, Vayssie C. A new approach to the bending properties of hair fibers. *J Cosmet Sci* 2001;**52**:355–68.
41. Gamez-Garcia M. Plastic yielding and fracture of human hair cuticles by cyclical torsion stresses. *J Cosmet Sci* 1999;**50**:69–77.
42. Feughelman M, Willis B. Mechanical extension of human hair and the movement of the cuticle. *J Cosmet Sci* 2001;**52**:185–93.
43. Schueller R, Romanowski P. Conditioning agents for hair and skin. *Cosmet Toilet* 1995;**110**:43–7.
44. Braida D, Dubief C, Lang G. Ceramide. A new approach to hair protection and conditioning. *Cosmet Toilet* 1994;**109**:49–57.
45. Rieger M. Surfactants in shampoos. *Cosmet Toilet* 1988;**103**:59.
46. Corbett JF. The chemistry of hair-care products. *J Soc Dyers Colour* 1976;**92**:285–303.
47. Allardice A, Gummo G. Hair conditioning: quaternary ammonium compounds on various hair types. *Cosmet Toilet* 1993;**108**: 107–9.
48. Allardice A, Gummo G. Hair conditioning. *Cosmet Toilet* 1993;**108**:107–9.
49. Ruetsch S, Kamath Y, Weigmann H. The role of cationic conditioning compounds in reinforcement of the cuticula. *J Cosmet Sci* 2003; **54**:63–83.
50. Idson B, Lee W. Update on hair conditioner ingredients. *Cosmet Toilet* 1983;**98**:41–6.
51. Dalton J, Allen G, Heard P *et al.* Advancements in spectroscopic and microscopic techniques for investigating the adsorption of conditioning polymers onto human hair. *J Cosmet Sci* 2000;**51**:275–87.
52. Finkelstein P. Hair conditioners. *Cutis* 1970; **6**:543–4.
53. Griesbach U, Klingels M, Horner V. Proteins: classic additives and actives for skin and hair care. *Cosmet Toilet* 1998;**113**:69–73.
54. Fox C. An introduction to the formulation of shampoos. *Cosmet Toilet* 1988;**103**:25–58.
55. Spoor HJ, Lindo SD. Hair processing and conditioning. *Cutis* 1974;**14**:689–94.
56. Swift J, Chahal S, Challoner N, Parfrey J. Investigations on the penetration of hydrolyzed wheat proteins into human hair by confocal laser-scanning fluorescence microscopy. *J Cosmet Sci* 2000;**51**:193–203.
57. Rosen M. Silicone Innovation for Hair Care. *GCI* 2002;37–9.
58. Ruiz M, Hernandez A, Llacer J, Gallardo V. Silicone chemistry. *Cosmet Toilet* 1998;**113**: 57–62.
59. Berthiaume M, Merrifield J, Riccio D. Effects of silicone pretreatment on oxidative hair damage. *J Soc Cosmet Chem* 1995;**46**: 231–45.
60. Reeth I, Caprasse V, Postiaux S, Starch M. Hair shine: correlation of instrumental and visual methods for measuring the effects of silicones. *IFSCC* 2001;**4**:21–6.

61. Starch M. Screening silicones for hair luster. *Cosmet Toilet* 1999;**114**:56–60.
62. Fox C. Hair care. *Cosmet Toilet* 1993;**108**:29–57.
63. Braida D, Dubief C, Lang G. Ceramide: a new approach to hair protection and conditioning. *Cosmet Toilet* 1994;**109**:49–57.
64. Bouillon C. Shampoos and hair conditioners. *Clin Dermatol* 1988;**6**:83–92.
65. Syed A, Ayoub H. Correlating porosity and tensile strength of chemically modified hair. *Cosmet Toilet* 2002;**117**:57–62.
66. Gao T, Bedell A. Ultraviolet damage on natural gray hair and its photoprotection. *J Cosmet Sci* 2001;**52**:103–18.
67. Georgalas A. Photoprotection for hair. *Cosmet Toilet* 1993;**108**:75–9.
68. Vanemon P. Photoprotection of human hair. *Cosmet Toilet* 1998;**113**:77–9.
69. Ruetsch S, Kamath Y, Weigmann H. Photodegradation of human hair: an SEM study. *J Cosmet Sci* 2000;**51**:103–25.
70. Ratnapandian S, Warner S, Kamath Y. Photodegradation of human hair. *J Cosmet Sci* 1998;**49**:309–20.
71. Arnoud R, Perbet G, Deflandre A, Lang G. ESR study of hair and melanin-keratin mixtures: the effects of temperature and light. *Int J Cosmet Sci* 1984;**6**:71–83.
72. Hoting E, Zimmerman M, Hocker H. Photochemical alterations in human hair. Part II. Analysis of melanin. *J Soc Cosmet Chem* 1995;**46**:181–90.
73. Jachowicz J. Hair damage and attempts to its repair. *J Soc Cosmet Chem* 1987;**38**:263–86.
74. Kirschenbaum L, Qu X, Borish E. Oxygen radicals from photoirradiated human hair: an ESR and fluorescence study. *J Cosmet Sci* 2000;**51**:169–82.
75. Holt LA, Milligan B. The formation of carbonyl groups during irradiation of wool and its relevance to photoyellowing. *Textile Res J* 1977;**47**:620–4.
76. Launer HF. Effect of light upon wool. IV. Bleaching and yellowing by sunlight. *Textile Res J* 1965;**35**:395–400.
77. Inglis AS, Lennox FG. Wool yellowing. IV. Changes in amino acid composition due to irradiation. *Textile Res J* 1963;**33**:431–5.
78. Tolgyesi E. Weathering of the hair. *Cosmet Toilet* 1983;**98**:29–33.
79. Ruetsch S, Kamath Y, Weigmann H. Photodegradation of human hair: an SEM study. *J Cosmet Sci* 2000;**51**:103–25.
80. Hoting E, Zimmerman M, Hocker H. Photochemical alterations in human hair. Part II. Analysis of melanin. *J Soc Cosmet Chem* 1995;**46**:181–90.
81. Milligan B, Tucker DJ. Studies on wool yellowing. Part III Sunlight yellowing. *Textile Res J* 1962;**32**:634.
82. Berth P, Reese G. Alteration of hair keratin by cosmetic processing and natural environmental influences. *J Soc Cosm Chem* 1964;**15**:659–66.
83. Gao T, Bedell A. Ultraviolet damage on natural gray hair and its photoprotection. *J Cosmet Sci* 2001;**52**:103–118.
84. Hoting E, Zimmerman M. Sunlight-induced modifications in bleached, permed, or dyed human hair. *J Soc Cosmet Chem* 1997;**48**:79–91.
85. Hoting E, Zimmerman M. Sunlight-induced modifications in bleached, permed, or dyed human hair. *J Soc Cosmet Chem* 1997;**48**:79–91.
86. Vanemon P. Photoprotection of human hair. *Cosmet Toilet* 1998;**113**:77–9.
87. Nacht S. Sunscreens and hair. *Cosmet Toilet* 1990;**105**:55–9.
88. Gonzenbach H, Johncock W, De Polo K *et al.* UV damage on human hair: a comparison study of 10 UV filters. *Cosmet Toilet* 1998;**113**:43–9.
89. Whittam JH. Hair care safety. In: Whittam JH, ed. *Cosmetic safety*. New York: Marcel Dekker, 1987:335–43.
90. Jachowicz J, Helioff M. Spatially resolved combing analysis. *J Soc Cosmet Chem* 1997;**48**:93–105.
91. Rollins TG: Traction folliculitis with hair casts and alopecia. *Am J Dis Child* 1961;**101**:639–40.
92. Scott DA. Disorders of the hair and scalp in blacks. *Dermatol Clin* 1988;**6**:387–95.
93. Rudolph RI, Klein AW, Decherd JW. Corn-row alopecia. *Arch Dermatol* 1973;**108**:134.
94. Morgan HV. Traction alopecia. *BMJ* 1960;**1**:115–117.
95. Slepyan AH. Traction alopecia. *Arch Dermatol* 1958;**78**:395–8.

96. Robbins CR. *Chemical and physical behavior of human hair*, 2nd edn. New York: Springer-Verlag, 1988:89–91.
97. McMullen R, Jachowicz J. Thermal degradation of hair. I. Effect of curling irons. *J Cosmet Sci* 1998;**49**:223–44.
98. Syed AN: Ethnic hair care. *Cosmet Toilet* 1993;**108**:99–107.
99. Grimes PE, Davis LT: Cosmetics in blacks. *Dermatol Clin* 1991;**9**:53–68.
100. LoPresti P, Papa DM, Kligman AM. Hot comb alopecia. *Arch Dermatol* 1968;**98**:234–8.
101. Sperling LC, Sau P. The follicular degeneration syndrome in black patients. *Arch Dermatol* 1992;**128**:68–74.

3 Hair grooming cosmetics

Hairstyles are in part dictated by the available technology in hairstyling products. The invention of hair gel virtually introduced a whole era of male fashion in the 1950s marked by slicked back stiff hair. This characteristic male hairstyle reminiscent of the movies *Grease* and *American Graffiti* would not have been possible without the discovery of hair gelling agents that made the hair stiff and shiny. A similar memorable era in female hairstyling was the 1960s bouffant beehive. This architectural hair wonder was made possible by the development of aerosol hairsprays based on newly discovered varnishes.

The current hairstyles of the millenium focus on the 'bed head' look and the attainment of perfectly 'spiked' hair. Formable hair waxes made possible through the development of polymers that soften at body temperature such that they can be reformed, yet provide a soft hold in the desired position, are responsible for creating the 'just got out of bed look.' The short spiked hair popular among teenaged boys is created by an updated high-hold version of the 1950s hair gel. All of this has been made possible by the ingenuity of the cosmetic chemist and hairstylists. The role of the physician is to understand how these products impact the hair and skin.[1] This section discusses the formulation and use of hairsprays, gels, waxes, mousses, pomades, brilliantines, oil sheen sprays, and curl activators (Table 3.1).

HAIRSPRAY

Hairspray is an aerosolized liquid applied to the hair following styling to maintain the hair in the desired position (Figure 3.1).[2,3] Hairsprays employ copolymers, such as polyvinylpyrrolidone (PVP), which add stiffness to the individual hairs and create temporary bonds between the hair shafts (Figure 3.2). PVP is a resin that is soluble in water and easily removed by shampooing; however, it is also able to absorb water. This means that the hairspray film will become sticky when mixed with perspiration, humidity, or precipitation. Also, the hair will no longer maintain the desired style. In order to make high-hold hairsprays, the PVP was mixed with vinyl acetate (VA) to form a new polymer (PVP/MA) (Figure 3.3). While vinyl acetate made the hairspray more resistant to water in the environment, it also made the hairspray harder to remove with shampooing.[4] This led to the development of other

Table 3.1 Hair grooming cosmetics

Styling product	Formulation	Application
Hairspray	Aerosolized spray polymer	Sprayed on a finished hairstyle
Hairstyling gel	Clear gel polymer	Rubbed with the hands onto towel-dried hair
Hair sculpturing gel	Clear gel higher concentration polymer	Rubbed with the hands onto towel-dried hair
Hair wax	Soft opaque formable wax	Massaged into dry hair shafts after softening in the palm
Hair mousse	Aerosolized polymer foam	Squirted onto the hand and dabbed through towel-dried hair
Pomade	Ointment of petrolatum	Combed with the hands through washed or unwashed hair
Brilliantine	Liquid oil	Massaged with the hands through washed or unwashed hair
Oil sheen spray	Aerosolized oil	Sprayed onto washed or unwashed hair
Curl activator	Clear glycerin gel	Massaged with the hands through washed or unwashed hair

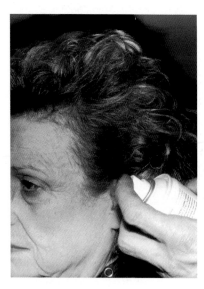

Figure 3.1
Hairspray application.

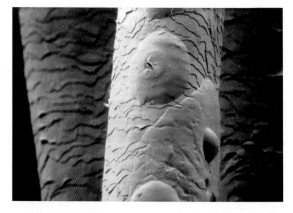

Figure 3.2
An electron micrograph of a regular-hold hairspray.

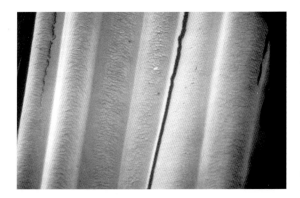

Figure 3.3
The appearance of a high-hold hairspray on the hair shafts.

copolymer resins of vinylmethylether and maleic acid hemiesters (PVP/MA) and copolymer resins of vinyl acetate and crotonic acid or dimethylhydantoin-formaldehyde.[5] The newest flexible-hold hairsprays that provide high hold with reduced stiffness may contain methacrylate copolymers, such as polyvinylpyrrolidone dimethylaminoethylmethacrylate (PVP/DMAEMA)[6,7] (Figures 3.4 and 3.5).

Even though the copolymer is the most important ingredient in hairspray, other ingredients must also be included to allow the aerosol spray to function.[8] These include plasticizers, humectants, solvents, and conditioners (Table 3.2).[9] This combination of ingredients is generally felt to be safe; however, there was some concern in the 1960s regarding inhalation of PVP/VA aerosolized particles.[10] After extensive animal testing, it was concluded that PVP resin did not provoke pulmonary lesions.[11,12] Nevertheless, persons who are predisposed to lung conditions or those with allergic tendencies should use hairspray products with care.[13] Hairsprays may be patch tested 'as is,' but should be allowed to dry thoroughly prior to occluding.

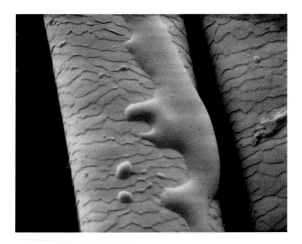

Figure 3.4
An electron micrograph of a flexible-hold hairspray.

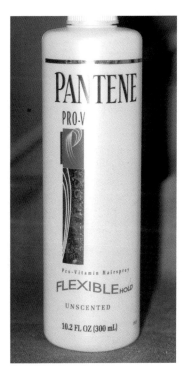

Figure 3.5
A commercially available flexible-hold pump hairspray.

Table 3.2 Hair spray formulation

Function	Sample ingredients
Copolymer	Polyvinylpyrrolidone and vinyl acetate (PVP/MA), vinylmethylether and maleic acid hemiesters (PVP/MA), polyvinylpyrrolidone and dimethylaminoethylmethacrylate (PVP/DMAEMA)
Plasticizer	Mineral oil, lanolin, castor oil, butyl palmitate
Humectant	Sorbitol, glycerol
Solvent	SD alcohol 40, isopropyl alcohol
Conditioner	Panthenol, plant proteins, hydrolyzed animal protein, quaternium-19

GEL

Hair gels are similar to hairsprays, except that they are squeezed from a tube rather than sprayed from a bottle. This product is applied to towel-dried, damp hair and distributed on the hair shafts by hand combing to form a thin film. If a small amount of gel is applied, the hair will have a natural look and feel. If a large amount is applied, the hair will have a wet 'spiky' look and a stiff feel. Hair gels contain the same PVP-type copolymers as hairsprays and offer enhanced hold, increased hair shine, and some conditioning (Figure 3.6).[14] Hair gels are available in two types: styling gels and sculpturing gels. Styling gels offer moderate hold while sculpturing gels offer strong hold, allowing the creation of gravity-defying hair styles (Figure 3.7). This is particularly important in persons with thinning hair, since the eye interprets hair thickness

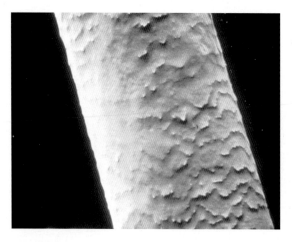

Figure 3.6
An electron micrograph demonstrating the polymer coating as it appears over a hair shaft.

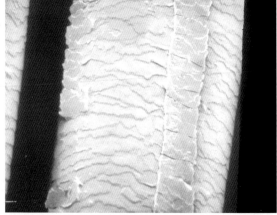

Figure 3.7
Electron micrograph of hair sculpturing gel on hair shaft.

by the hair elevation over the crown and the lateral displacement at the sides of the head.[15] Hair gels can hold the hair away from the scalp, creating the illusion of fullness.[16] They may be patch tested 'as is,' but should be allowed to dry thoroughly prior to occlusion with a patch.

WAX

Hair waxes are relatively new products designed to add increased hold to hair. They too rely on polymers, but the polymers are designed to soften at body temperature. Also, the polymers can be easily reformed, providing a styling product that can be reshaped frequently yet allow the hair to remain in position. These are the products that allow the 'bed head' look where the hair stands straight on end away from the scalp, but has a rather greasy appearance (Figure 3.8). These products are scooped from a can by the fingers and allowed to soften in the palm prior to application. They are massaged along the length of the hair shafts to provide an even thin coating. Hair waxes are

basically popular among young persons with very short hair.

MOUSSE

Hair mousses are unique styling products in that they are released as foam from an aerosolized can. The mousse is applied in the same manner as a hair gel to towel-dried hair. It can also be applied to dry hair to create a wet spiky look. Hair mousse yields a lighter copolymer application and does not provide as strong a hold as gel formulations. It also produces less flaking and stickiness under moist conditions. Men generally prefer this product.

Hair mousses are based on the same copolymers as hairsprays and hair gels. In addition, they may contain glossing and conditioning agents and can be colored to provide either natural or unnatural highlights. For example, persons with less than 15% gray hair can use colored mousse with brown or auburn hues to blend gray hair. Unnatural colors such as yellow, green, red, orange, purple, and blue are also available.

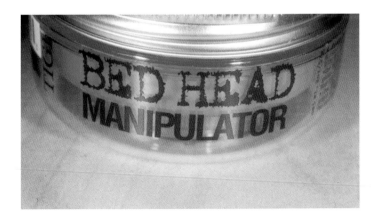

Figure 3.8
An example of a commercially available hair wax.

The color is temporary and removed with one shampooing unless applied to chemically treated hair.

POMADES

Hair pomades are designed to straighten, condition, moisturize, and add shine to kinky hair found in African-American persons (Table 3.3). Pomades, also known as cream brilliantines, are anhydrous products containing petrolatum, waxes, lanolin, and vegetable or mineral oils[17] (Figure 3.9). Treatment pomades may also contain sulfur, vitamins, or tar derivatives to minimize the recurrence and symptoms of dandruff or seborrheic dermatitis (Figure 3.10). The thick pomade ointment helps to minimize combing friction in tightly kinked hair, preventing hair breakage with styling through lubrication. The petrolatum also prevents water evaporation, a common unwanted side effect of hair straightening, discussed in detail in Chapter 6. The pomade can also act

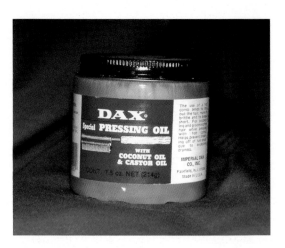

Figure 3.9
A commercially marketed hair pomade.

as a styling product to allow the hair to remain close to the scalp with some curl reduction.

One possible problem associated with pomade use is pomade acne, as reported by Plewig et al.[18] Pomade acne is comedonal acne along the hairline frequently seen in patients using olive oil-containing

Table 3.3 Black hair styling products

Styling product	Type	Formulation	Function
Pomade	Cream	Petrolatum, wax, lanolin, mineral oil, vegetable oil	Moisturize hair, add shine, decrease breakage, aid in straightening hair
Brilliantine	Liquid	Vegetable oils, mineral oil, silicone	Moisturize hair, add shine
Oil sheen spray	Aerosol	Vegetable oils, mineral oil, silicone	Moisturize hair, add shine
Gel curl activator	Gel	Glycerin	Moisturize hair, add shine

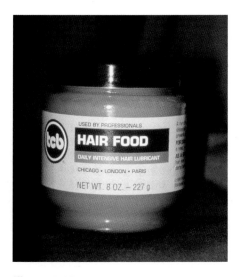

Figure 3.10
A sulfur-based pomade.

OIL SHEEN SPRAY

Hairsprays for kinky hair must contain a high concentration of conditioners. One unique form of hairspray for African-American hair is the oil sheen spray (Figure 3.11). This is an aerosolized oil, for example containing mineral oil and silicone, which is sprayed onto the hair on a daily basis to moisturize and decrease combing friction. It may also contain steartrimonium hydrolyzed animal protein and a difatty cationic amino acid derivative for additional shine and moisturization.

CURL ACTIVATORS

The previously discussed pomades, brilliantines, and oil sheen sprays are designed

pomades.[18] The petrolatum and mineral oil are not the cause of the acne. It is the presence of comedogenic olive oil that is problematic. Thus, individuals who are prone to the formation of acne should avoid hair products containing olive oil and other vegetable oils.

BRILLIANTINE

Pomades are ointments while hair brilliantines are liquids. Liquid brilliantines are popular for maintaining natural, kinky hairstyles. These products allow ease of styling and provide shine without causing an oil build-up. Traditionally they contain mineral and vegetable oils and may be comedogenic.[19,20] Newer formulations contain silicone to add lubricity, castor oil to aid in manageability, and soluble glycoprotein to maintain proper moisture balance and enhance shine.[21]

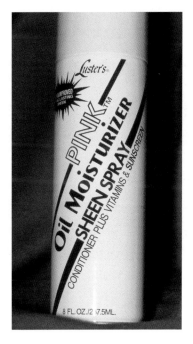

Figure 3.11
An oil sheen spray.

for straightened or relaxed hair; however, these products are not suitable for use on kinky hair that has undergone permanent waving to create soft ringlets. The permanent waving of African-American hair to create soft curls is known as a 'Jheri curl,' after the name of the company that popularized the hairstyle. This hairstyle requires moisturization, but the heavy ointments and oils would prevent the curls from forming. Gel curl activators were developed specifically for this ringlet hairstyle (Figure 3.12). They are based on glycerin, which functions as a humectant to attract water to the hair shafts. These clear gels are scooped from a jar and stroked through the hair prior to styling, but do not moisturize quite as well as the traditional pomades. Recently, they have fallen out of popularity because glycerin leaves the hair sticky and also attracts dirt, requiring frequent shampooing. Unfortunately, the glycerin also was not water-resistant, meaning that the entire hairstyle had to be redesigned with each shampooing.

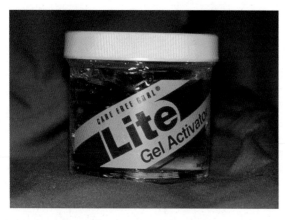

Figure 3.12
A gel curl activator.

REFERENCES

1. McMullen R, Jachowicz J. Optical properties of hair: effect of treatments on luster as quantified by image analysis. *J Cosmet Sci* 2003;**54**:335–51.
2. Jachowicz J, Yao K. Dynamic hairspray analysis. I. Instrumentation and preliminary results. *J Soc Cosmet Chem* 1996;**47**:73–84.
3. Guth J, Russo J, Kay T, King N, Beaven R. Addressing the low VOC hair spray issue. *Cosmet Toilet* 1993;**108**:97–103.
4. Wells FV, Lubowe II: hair grooming aids, part III. *Cutis* 1978;**22**:407–25.
5. Pavlichko J. Aqueous dispersion hair-spray resin. *Cosmet Toilet* 1995;**110**:63–7.
6. Zviak C. *The science of hair care*. New York: Marcel Dekker, 1986,153–65.
7. Stutsman MJ. Analysis of hair fixatives. In: Newburger's manual of cosmetic analysis, 2nd edn. Washington, DC: Association of Official Analytical Chemists, 1977:72.
8. Jachowicz J, Yao K. Dynamic hairspray analysis. II. Effect of polymer, hair type, and solvent composition. *J Cosmet Sci* 2001;**52**: 281–95,
9. Lochhead RY, Hemker WJ, Castaneda JY. Hair care gels. *Cosmet Toilet* 1987;**102**:89–100.
10. Oteri R, Tazi M, Walls E, Kosiek J. Formulating hairsprays for new air quality regulations. *Cosmet Toilet* 1991;**106**:29–34.
11. Zviak C. *The science of hair care*. New York: Marcel Dekker, 1986:167–8.
12. Wells FV, Lubowe II. Hair grooming aids, part IV. *Cutis* 1978;**22**:557–62.
13. Wilkinson JB, Moore RJ. *Harry's cosmeticology*. New York: Chemical Publishing, 1982: 481–3.
14. Wood C, Nguyen-Kim S, Hoessel P. A new dimension in hairstyling – VP/methacrylamide/vinyl imidazole copolymer. *Cosmet Toilet* 2003;**118**:59–66.
15. Clarke J, Robbins CR, Reich C. Influence of hair volume and texture on hair body of tresses. *J Soc Cosmet Chem* 1991;**42**:341–52.

16. Rushton DH, Kingsley P, Berry NL, Black S. Treating reduced hair volume in women. *Cosmet Toilet* 1993;**108**:59–62.

17. Goode ST. Hair pomades. *Cosmet Toilet* 1979; **94**:71–4.

18. Plewig G, Fulton JE, Kligman AM. Pomade acne. *Arch Dermatol* 1970;**101**:580–4.

19. Balsam MS, Sagarin E. Hair grooming prepa-rations. In: *Cosmetics: Science and technology*, 2nd edn., New York: Wiley-Interscience, 1972:119–23.

20. Rele A, Mohile R. Effect of coconut oil on prevention of hair damage. Part 1. *J Cosmet Sci* 1999;**50**:327–39,

21. Wells FV, Lubowe II. Hair grooming aids, Part II. *Cutis* 1978;**22**:270–301.

4   Hair coloring techniques

Hair coloring is a technique used by both men and women for altering the natural hair color or camouflaging the presence of gray hair (Figure 4.1).[1]   The hair color can be changed until the next shampooing, for 8–12 shampooings, or permanently.[2] It can be dyed darker than the original hair color or lightened. This invention has added a whole new dimension to hair cosmetics and created a huge at-home hair dye and salon industry.

Even though henna and indigo have been used to color hair for over 3000 years, modern synthetic organic chemistry has made the twentieth century the era of hair color. The whole hair coloring industry began when Hoffman in 1863 noticed that para-phylenediamine produced a brown-black coloration when oxidized. But, the transfer of knowledge was slow in the late 1800s and it was not until 1907 that Eugene Schueller marketed the first commercial brand of hair color. He was a chemist and the founder of L'Oreal, still a leader in hair coloring technology today. Originally, hair coloring was limited to the professional salon, but in 1950 the first home-use hair dye was introduced.

Several companies, besides L'Oreal have dominated the US hair coloring market:

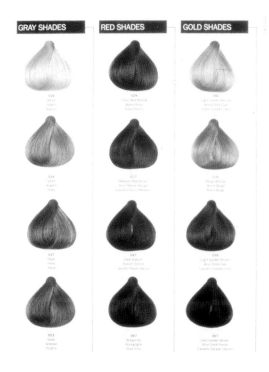

Figure 4.1
Tremendous color variation can be achieved through the use of hair coloring cosmetics.

Clairol, founded in 1931, and Roux, also founded in 1931. Clairol was founded by Lawrence Gelb who purchased the original hair coloring formulas from Dr Friedreich Klein, a German chemist, for $25,000. By 1938, the sales of Clairol hair color had reached $1 million. The first hair color introduced by Clairol was called 'Instant Clairol' and was reformulated in 1950 as 'Miss Clairol Haircolor Bath.' Further advances were made possible by the development of semipermanent dyes, dyes that washed out after 6–10 shampoos, and this resulted in the launch of 'Clairol Loving Care.'

In order to understand hair dyeing, it is first necessary to undertake a brief discussion of the natural pigments contained in the hair shaft. Pigment comprises less than 3% of the fiber mass of hair, yet is one of the most important hair cosmetic aspects.[3] Three pigment types produce the tremendous variety of color seen in human hair: eumelanins, pheomelanins, and oxymelanins. Eumelanins are insoluble polymers accounting for the brown and black hues, consisting mainly of 5,6-dihydroxyindole with lesser amounts of 5,6-dihydroxyindole-2-carboxylic acid (Figure 4.2). Pheomelanins are soluble polymers accounting for the yellow to red hues containing 10–12% sulfur and 1,4-benzothiazinylalanine (Figure 4.3). Eumelanin contains fewer sulfurs than pheomelanin.[4] A lesser pigment, known as oxymelanin, is yellow or reddish in color and probably represents bleached eumelanin pigment arising from partial oxidative cleavage of 5,6-dihydroxyindole units. Oxymelanin is distinct in that it contains no sulfur.[5] Hair dyes attempt to mimic these pigments in reproducing a natural appearing hair color (Figure 4.4).

The principal use for hair dyeing is to cover gray hair. The mechanism of graying is not totally understood, however. It is thought that the death of some melanocytes within the hair-melanocyte unit triggers a chain reaction resulting in the death of the rest of the unit melanocytes in a relatively short period.[6] A possible mechanism of

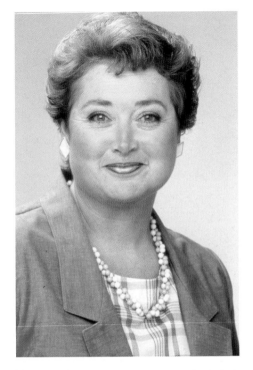

Figure 4.2
Eumelanin dominance creating brunette hair.

death is the accumulation of a toxic intermediate metabolite, such as dopaquinone.[7]

Several different types of hair dye cosmetics have been developed: gradual, temporary, semipermanent, and permanent (Figure 4.5). Approximately 65% of the hair dye market purchases are for permanent hair colorings, 20% for semipermanent colorings, and 15% for the remaining types. Each type will be discussed in detail (Table 4.1).

GRADUAL

Gradual hair dyes, also known as metallic or progressive hair dyes, require repeated

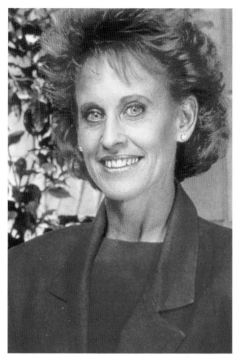

Figure 4.3
Pheomelanin dominance creating red
hair.

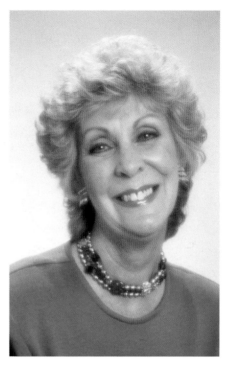

Figure 4.4
Blond hair created through synthetic
hair dye pigments.

application to result in gradual darkening of the hair shaft (Grecian Formula for Men and Grecian Formula for Women, Combe International, White Plains, NY, USA) (Figure 4.6). This product will change the hair color from gray to yellow-brown to black over a period of weeks.[8] There is no control over the final color of the hair, only the depth of color, and lightening is not possible. These products employ water-soluble metal salts which are deposited on the hair shaft in the form of oxides, suboxides, and sulfides. The most common metal used is lead, but silver, copper, bismuth, nickel, iron, manganese, and cobalt have also been used. In the United States, 2–3% solutions of lead acetate or nitrate are used to dye the hair while 1–2% solutions of silver nitrate are used to dye eyelashes and eyebrows.[9]

The popularity of gradual hair dyes is due to their low cost and the ability to perform the dyeing procedures at home without the assistance of a professional operator. They must be properly applied, however, or poor color quality, stiff, brittle, and dull hair may result. In addition, the trace metals left on the hair do not allow predictable results when combined with other dyeing or permanent waving procedures. The metal can cause breakdown of the hydrogen peroxide in bleaching or permanent waving products, resulting in rupture of the hair shaft. Hair that has been treated with a gradual hair colorant must therefore grow out before other dyeing or waving procedures are used to guarantee an optimal result.[10]

This type of hair coloring is most popular among men who wish to only blend their

Table 4.1 Types of hair dye

Hair dye type	Chemical reaction	Anticipated end result	Duration of effect	Advantages	Disadvantages
Gradual	Deposition of metal salts	Gradual brown hair darkening	Requires continuous application	Inexpensive, easy to apply	Cannot be combined with other chemical hair processing
Temporary	Acid textile dyes	Blending of hair tones	One shampoo exposure	Short-lived, inexpensive	May rub off on clothing or run with water exposure
Semi-permanent: vegetable	Henna with metal salts	Reddish hues to hair	4–6 shampoo exposures	Low incidence of allergenicity	Leave hair somewhat harsh
Semi-permanent: textile	Textile dyes	Tone hair, minimally cover gray	4–6 shampoo exposures	Add color highlights	Short-lived color
Demi-permanent	Deeper penetrating textile dyes	Tone hair, minimally cover gray	10–12 shampoo exposures	Longer-lasting with no obvious hair grow-out	Cannot completely cover gray
Permanent	Oxidation/reduction reaction	Darken hair color, cover gray	Permanent	Excellent coverage of gray hair	Color is permanent
One-step bleaching	Oxidation/reduction reaction	Lighten hair color, cover gray	Permanent	Achieve light blond hair shades	Damaging to hair
Two-step bleaching	Oxidative alkaline reaction	Dramatically lighten hair color, cover gray	Permanent	Achieve dramatic hair color lightening	Very damaging to hair

gray hair and effect hair color darkening gradually. Men also tend to cut their hair frequently, which removes the hair that may have been damaged by repeated use of the metallic dye. Continued application is necessary to maintain the desired color, which can make the hair shaft cosmetically unacceptable with time. Men also are not as likely as women to undergo permanent waving procedures. Therefore, gradual hair dyes are

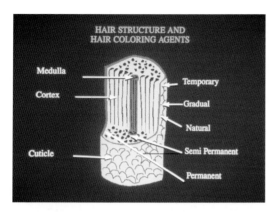

Figure 4.5
The penetration of each of the different hair dyes into the hair shaft is demonstrated.

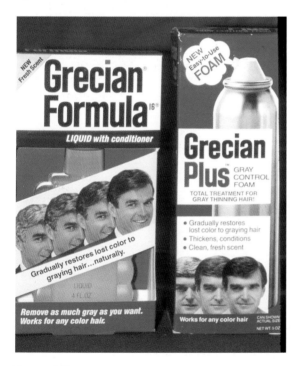

Figure 4.6
An example of a commercially available gradual hair dye.

not appropriate for female patients who desire more color darkening than the product can provide and who are likely to undergo permanent waving.[11]

TEMPORARY

Temporary hair coloring agents comprise only 3% of the hair coloring market and are removed in one shampooing.[12] They are used to add a slight tint, brighten a natural shade, or improve an existing dyed shade. Their particle size is too large to penetrate through the cuticle, accounting for their temporary nature.[13] However, the dye can be easily rubbed off the hair shaft and can run onto clothing if the hair gets wet from rain or perspiration. Temporary hair dyes do not damage the hair shaft and may be used by persons who are allergic to paraphenylenediamine. These dyes are most popular among elderly women who wish to achieve platinum hair. This is accomplished by adding a bluish or purplish temporary rinse to the hair after shampooing to cover yellow hues in the hair created by small amounts of remaining eumelanin or pheomelanin.

Male and female adolescents may use temporary hair colorants to create blue, green, red, or purple hair for a weekend party (Figure 4.7). They can also be applied to selected areas of the scalp to create multicolored hair. These hair effects are created by temporary hair dye sprays, mousses, or gels. The newest trend has been to add glitter to the temporary hair dyes to create iridescent hair. The United States gymnasts popularized this effect in the recent summer Olympics. Hair glitter can contribute to scalp pruritus and can cause corneal abrasion if accidentally introduced into the eye.

There are several formulations of temporary dyes: liquid, mousse, and gel. Liquid temporary hair colorants are also referred to as 'hair rinses' since they are frequently applied in the shower following shampooing, with the excess dyestuff removed by rinsing. They contain acid dyes of the same type used to dye wool fabrics and belong to the following chemical classes: azo, anthraquinone, triphenylmethane, phenzainic,

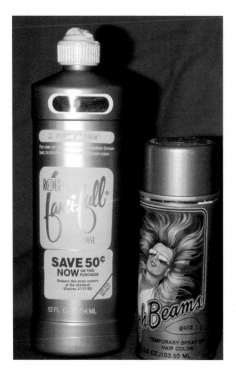

Figure 4.7
Party colors can be achieved with
temporary hair colorings.

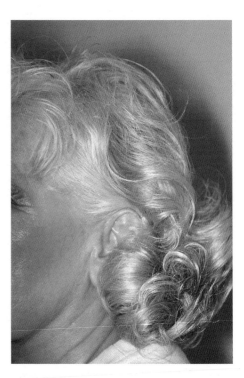

Figure 4.8
An example of hair dyed purple while
trying to brighten gray hair.

xanthenic, or benzoquinoneimine.[14] These
dyes are known as FDC and DC blues,
greens, reds, oranges, yellows and violets.
No damage is imparted to the hair shaft by
these dyes, making them appropriate for
men and women of all hair types.

The liquid rinse formulation is most popular, especially among mature patients with
gray hair who wish to remove undesirable
yellow tones and achieve a purer platinum
color (Figure 4.8). A sample product for this
purpose may contain a 0.001% concentration of methylene blue, acid violet 6B and
water-soluble nigrosine in an aqueous
preparation. Temporary hair colorants are
recommended for mature patients who style
their hair once weekly, since the dye must be
reapplied with each shampooing.

Mousse formulations of temporary hair
colorants are available in both natural and
party colors. They are applied following
shampooing to towel-dried hair and are not
removed. Because the coloring agent is dis-
persed in a styling polymer, such as
polyvinylpyrrolidone/vinyl acetate (PVP/VA),
the mousse serves both as a styling agent
and temporary colorant. This product may
be used to add highlights or blend gray hair
in brunette patients with less than 15% gray
hair. Mousse temporary coloring agents are
ideal for the female patient with minimal
bitemporal graying. These products are also
available in party colors such as yellow,
orange, blue, green, purple, and red, which
can be used to create special multicolored
effects.

Gel formulations of temporary hair colorants are identical to mousse formulations,
except that they are packaged as a gel in a
tube rather than a foam released from an

aerosol can. Gel temporary hair colorants also combine a styling aid with coloring; however, the hold provided by the gel is generally superior to that provided by the mousse. These products are only available in party colors, with some lines including a hair glitter.[15]

Temporary hair coloring agents should be used with care in patients with damaged or chemically treated hair because the hair shaft has increased porosity due to loss of the cuticular scale. The porous hair shafts allow entrance of the color molecules into the hair shaft, rendering them more permanent. Under these conditions, it may take more than one shampooing to remove the color.

An understanding of temporary hair dyes is useful to the dermatologist, since these textile dyes do not further damage the hair shaft. Occasionally, a patient may present who is dismayed with the undesirable color of her hair following an unsuccessful dyeing procedure. Many of these patients are anxious to redye their hair to a different shade. Unfortunately, repeat dyeing procedures undertaken in a short period of time may result in even more unpredictable color outcomes and irreversibly damaged, weakened hair. Temporary hair colorings can be recommended to this distraught patient as a way of achieving a better hair color, while waiting for fading of the undesirable color and new growth.

SEMIPERMANENT

Semipermanent hair coloring accounts for only 10% of the current hair care market. Table 4.2 lists the names of some of the currently marketed products as a reference for the dermatologist. These products can be purchased in drug stores and mass merchandisers (WalMart, Target, Kmart, etc.)

and are not formulated for professional salon use. They are designed for use on natural, unbleached hair to cover gray, add highlights, or rid hair of unwanted tones.[16]

Semipermanent dyes are retained in the hair shaft by weak polar and Van der Waals attractive forces, thus lasting through 6–10 shampooings.[17] Usually, 10–12 dyes are mixed to obtain the desired shade.[18] Semipermanent dyes produce tone-on-tone coloring rather than effecting drastic color changes, so their role is actually in toning rather than dyeing hair (Figure 4.9). The less color change required by the patient, the more satisfied he or she will be with the semipermanent dye result. Semipermanent dyes are best suited for patients with less than 30% gray hair who want to restore their natural color.[19] This is done by selecting a dye color that is lighter than the natural hair color since the dye will penetrate both the gray and the nongray hairs, resulting in an increased darkening of the nongray hairs. It is not possible to lighten hair with semipermanent dyes, since they do not contain hydrogen peroxide, nor is it possible to darken hair more than three shades beyond the patient's natural hair color. Thus, in the cosmetic industry, semipermanent dyes are known as suitable only for staying 'on shade.'

Table 4.2 Semipermanent hair coloring products: home-use products

Product name	Product type	Manufacturer
Avantage	Lotion	L'Oreal
Loving Care	Lotion	Clairol
Scala	Lotion	Wella
PolyColor	Aerosol foam	Henkel

Note: There are no professional salon semipermanent hair coloring products. Source: GCI, *The century of hair color*, JF Corbett, pp. 22–9, September 2001.

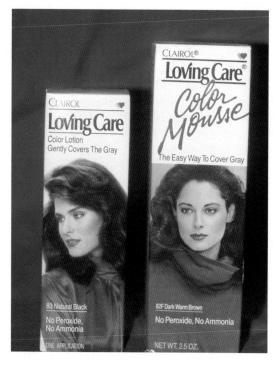

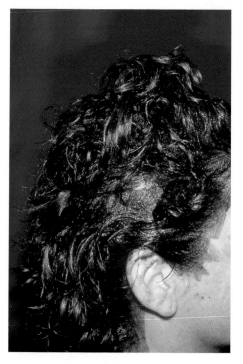

Figure 4.9
An example of a home-use semipermanent
hair coloring product.

Figure 4.10
The appearance of a semipermanent
dye on the hair.

There are several different types of semipermanent hair dyes based on the deriva-
tion of the dye. These include textile dyes,
vegetable dyes, and synthetic hair stains.
Each variety is discussed.

Textile dyes

Semipermanent hair colorings derived from
textile dyes are popular with both men and
women. Since human hair is basically a textile, dyes for wool and natural fiber cloths
are well suited for adaptation to hair dyeing.
The formulation of a typical semipermanent
textile-derived hair dye is dyes (nitroani-
lines, nitrophenylenediamines, nitroamino-

phenols, azos, anthraquinones), alkalizing
agent, solvent, surfactant, thickener, fragrance and water.[17] These dyes are commonly available as shampoos and mousses.
The shampoo-in process is most popular for
home use. The dyestuff is combined with an
alkaline detergent shampoo to promote hair
shaft swelling so that the dye can minimally
penetrate the hair shaft. Thickeners and
foam stabilizers are added so that the dye
will remain on the scalp and not run into the
eyes. The mousse formula incorporates the
dyestuff in an aerosolized foam. Both products are applied to wet, freshly shampooed
hair and are rinsed in 20–40 minutes (Figure
4.10). Semipermanent dyes can become
more permanent if applied to porous,
chemically treated hair.

Vegetable dyes

The very first hair dye ever developed historically was a vegetable dye known as henna. Henna is a plant that was used by the third dynasty of Egypt 4000 years ago to add red hues to their naturally brunette hair. The Egyptians mixed the henna plant, botanically known as *Lawsonia alba*, with hot water to make a paste. The paste was placed on the head for several hours to produce a characteristic orange-red hair color. Henna is a semipermanent dye because minimal cuticle penetration occurs allowing removal of the dye in 4–6 shampooings. The leaves of the henna plant contain a natural acidic naphthoquinone dye. More recently, henna has been combined with metallic salts to produce what is termed a 'compound henna', to provide a wider range of colors (Figure 4.11). These are the same metallic salts that were discussed previously under the gradual dye section.

Today, synthetic henna-type products have replaced natural henna dyes with dye shades ranging from auburn to blond to gray. These synthetic henna products combine a conditioning agent with the dye, but they are still powders mixed with water to form a paste that remains in contact with the hair for 40 minutes. Hennas can be used for darkening, but not lightening, of the original hair color. Natural hennas are inferior to synthetic hennas because they leave the hair stiff and brittle after repeated applications. Henna has not been reported to cause allergic contact dermatitis when used as a hair dye.

It is worth mentioning one additional unique historical vegetable hair dye that is distinct from henna. This dye is derived from black walnut tree leaves and was used in the south by women who wanted to darken their gray hair. This vegetable dye is able to darken gray hair without the use of allergenic paraphenylenediamine, which is found in virtually all permanent hair dyes. Black walnut hair dye (Herbasol, Cosmetochem USA) can be safely used to produce a deep brownish-black hair color in patients who are allergic to paraphenylenediamine. A more detailed discussion of hair dye allergy can be found later in this section (page 113).

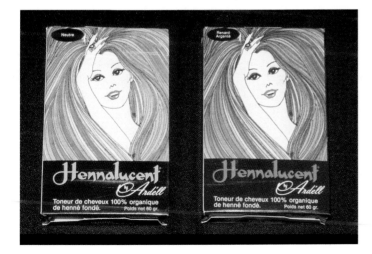

Figure 4.11
An example of modern henna hair coloring.

Synthetic stains

A newer type of semipermanent hair coloring is hair stain. Hair stain is a synthetic polymer, usually in unnatural shades such as red, blue, purple, or yellow, that imparts a hue or highlight to the hair (Cellophanes, Sebastian). For example, brunette hair with a red stain will have a reddish glow or blond hair with a yellow stain will have a yellow glow. The stain appears transparent so that it blends with the underlying hair color. The stain does not cover, but only tones. If heat is added to the staining process, the stain is more resistant to shampoo removal and if both heat and hydrogen peroxide are added to the staining process, the stain can penetrate the hair shaft deeply and become permanent.

DEMIPERMANENT

A newer form of hair coloring that is longer-lasting than semipermanent dyes, but still not permanent, is known as demipermanent hair coloring. Demipermanent dyes are replacing semipermanent dyes and are available in both home-use and professional salon use formulations (Table 4.3). They are longer-lasting, usually remaining through 10–12 shampooings, and have the advantage of longevity without sharp color contrast with new growth, a characteristic of permanent hair dyes.

These products are packaged for both men and women, with the newest introduction being the use of adolescent male models on some boxes. Demipermanent dyes do not lighten hair, but are used to primarily add red highlights to brunette hair. Most commonly they are used to give the hair a burgundy hue, not attainable naturally due to the presence of only eumelanins and

Table 4.3 Demipermanent hair coloring products

Product name	Product type	Manufacturer
Home-use products		
Castings	Lotion	L'Oreal
Natural instincts	Lotion	Clairol
Professional salon products		
Color Touch	Lotion	Wella
Complements	Cream	Clairol
Second Nature	Lotion	Clairol

Source: GCI, *The century of hair color*, JF Corbett, pp. 22–9, September 2001.

pheomelanins with brown and yellow colors. Burgundy hair requires the additional introduction of blue pigments into the hair shaft.

Demipermanent dyes are not as damaging to the hair shaft as permanent hair dyes, but may contain paraphylenediamine and thus may possibly cause allergic contact dermatitis in sensitized individuals.

PERMANENT

Permanent hair coloring is the most popular hair coloring technique on the market today, accounting for 85% of hair dyes sold for both professional salon and home use (Table 4.4). Three out of every four dollars spent on hair dyeing in the United States is for some type of permanent hair dye. Their popularity is due to tremendous color variety, most product lines contain 20 shades, and the ability to both lighten and darken hair (Figure 4.12). Permanent hair coloring is so named because the dyestuff penetrates the hair shaft to the cortex and forms large color

Table 4.4 Permanent hair coloring products

Product name	Product type	Manufacturer
Home-use products		
Bigen	Powder/lotion	Hoyu
ColorStay	Lotion	Revlon
Feria	Gel	L'Oreal
Hydrience	Gel	Clairol
Kao Hair Color	Lotion	Kao
Nice 'n Easy	Lotion	Clairol
Poly Color	Lotion	Henkel
Preference	Lotion	L'Oreal
Revitalique	Lotion	Clairol
Miss Clairol	Lotion	Clairol
Professional salon products		
Complements	Cream	Clairol
Fancitone	Lotion	Roux
Igora	Cream	Schwarzkopf
Koleston	Cream	Wella
Top Chic	Cream	Goldwell
Miss Clairol	Lotion	Clairol

Source: GCI, *The century of hair color*, JF Corbett, pp. 22–9, September 2001.

molecules that cannot be removed by shampooing.[20]

Permanent dyes have been embraced by mature men and women to cover gray and by adolescent boys and girls to lighten hair. Redyeing is necessary every 4–6 weeks, as new growth, known in the cosmetic industry as 'roots,' appears at the scalp. This is no longer considered a major disadvantage of permanent hair dyeing since multicolored hair has become fashionable. The Clairol advertising campaign of the 1960s that asked 'Does she or doesn't she?' challenged others to determine if the woman was a hair dye user. Now, adults and adolescent males and females seem proud to sport locks of a new color every other week. The use of permanent hair dyes is no longer a well kept secret.

Chemistry

Permanent hair coloring is so named because the dyestuff penetrates the hair shaft to the cortex and forms large color molecules that cannot be removed by shampooing.[20] This type of hair coloring does not contain dyes, but rather colorless dye precursors that chemically react with hydrogen

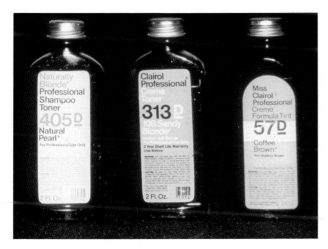

Figure 4.12
An example of permanent hair colorings for professional salon use.

peroxide inside the hair shaft to produce colored molecules.[21] The process entails the use of primary intermediates (p-phenylene-diamines, p-toluenediamine, p-aminophenols) which undergo oxidation with hydrogen peroxide. These reactive intermediates are then exposed to couplers (resorcinol, 1-naphthol, m-aminophenol, etc.) to result in a wide variety of indo dyes. These indo dyes can produce shades from blond to brown to black with highlights of gold to red to orange. Variations in the concentration of hydrogen peroxide and the chemicals selected for the primary intermediates and couplers produce this color selection.[22] Red is produced by using nitroparaphenylenediamine alone or in combination with mixtures of para-aminophenol with meta-phenylenediamine, alphanaphthol or 1,5-dihydroxynaphthalene. Yellow is produced by mixtures of orthoaminophenol, ortho-phenylenediamine and nitro-ortho-phenylenediamine. Blue has no single oxidation dye intermediate and is produced by combinations of paraphenylenediamine, phenylenediamine, methyltoluylenediamine or 2,4 diaminoanisol.[23]

Permanent dyeing allows shades to be obtained that are both lighter and darker than the patient's original hair color. Higher concentrations of hydrogen peroxide can bleach melanin, thus the oxidizing step functions both in color production and bleaching. Due to the use of hydrogen peroxide in the formation of the new color molecules, hair dyes must be adjusted so that hair lightening is not produced with routine dyeing.[24] However, hydrogen peroxide cannot remove sufficient melanin alone to lighten dark brown or black hair to blond hair. Boosters, such as ammonium persulfate or potassium sulfate, must be added to achieve great degrees of color lightening. The boosters must be left in contact with the hair for 1–2 hours for an optimal result. Nevertheless, individuals with dark hair who choose to dye their hair a light blond color will notice the appearance of reddish hues with time. This is due to the inability of the peroxide/booster system to completely remove reddish pheomelanin pigments, which are more resistant to removal than brownish eumelanin pigments.

Application techniques

Permanent hair dye can be applied at home or in a professional salon. Home permanent dye products can be purchased to lighten or darken the hair by three shades while salon products can achieve any color of the rainbow desired. Products that lighten the hair contain ammonia and hydrogen peroxide, thus bleaching and dyeing the hair in one step. A more detailed discussion of hair bleaching is presented on page 109. This section will present the application details for both home and salon use dye products with illustrations demonstrating salon application.

Permanent hair dyes for home use are sold as two bottles containing colorless liquid within a kit consisting of vinyl gloves and instructions. One bottle contains the dye precursors in an alkaline soap or synthetic detergent base and the other contains a stabilized solution of hydrogen peroxide. The two bottles are combined immediately prior to use and must be shaken vigorously to thoroughly mix the ingredients. This begins the oxidation/reduction reaction and the color of the hair dye begins to emerge. The dye must be applied immediately to dry unwashed hair and cannot be saved for later use. Following application, the dye precursors and hydrogen peroxide diffuse into the hair shaft cortex where the chemical reaction occurs. The dye is left in contact with the hair for 25–40 minutes, depending on the color selected and whether the hair has been previously chemically treated.

If the hair has been dyed previously, the dye is only applied to the new growth at the scalp initially and then combed through the ends of the hair for the last 10 minutes. This is due to the fact that previously dyed hair has a damaged cuticle and the dye will penetrate more rapidly. If the hair dye is left on new growth and previously dyed hair for the same length of time, the previously dyed hair will be a darker shade. The ability of a hair dye to color the hair is known in the salon industry as 'grab.' If the ends of the hair shafts are badly damaged, then a 'filler' is used to prevent the distal hair shafts from dyeing darker than the proximal hair shafts. This filler is applied prior to the dyeing process.

Once the dye has been left on the hair for the desired amount of time, it is thoroughly rinsed with water until the water runs clean. The hair dye must be removed from the skin and hair, since it will dye any protein. Seborrheic keratoses on the scalp will also dye, much to the dismay of elderly patients. Following rinsing, the hair is shampooed with a special conditioner. The dye induces cuticle swelling, which must be reversed to prevent excessive hair damage. The conditioner is applied to the hair and left on for 5 minutes followed by drying and styling.

Even though permanent hair dye is labeled 'permanent,' it is removed from the hair shaft with water contact. The newly created color molecules can diffuse out of the hair shaft, especially with frequent washing with a harsh shampoo. For this reason, special mild surfactant shampoos have been created to minimize the amount of dye removed. Nevertheless, some dye is lost with each water contact, accounting for a phenomenon known as 'color drift.' The dyed hair color tends to lighten with time and develop red tones. This red color shift is known as 'hair brassiness.' It occurs because the brown eumelanins are more susceptible to removal from the hair shaft than the red

pheomelanins. Thus, in hair that was dyed from light brown to dark brown, the brown colors are lost with shampooing leaving the natural pheomelanins behind. This increases the red hair tones, giving the hair a redder appearance than when it was first dyed. This same 'brassiness' occurs with blond hair that tends to lose the yellow colors with shampooing also developing red hues from the resistant natural pheomelanins. This brassiness used to be considered undesirable, yet adolescents now intentionally attempt to dye their brown hair blonde to create these unusual red tones.

It sometimes becomes necessary to cover undesirable brassiness or other unwanted hair tones until the hair can be redyed. Semipermanent hair colorings may be used for this purpose. These special dyes are known as 'drabbers.' Examples of drabbers are: resorcinol to yield dark green to brown colors, pyrocatechol to yield deep gray, pyrogallol to yield gold, alphanaphthol to yield bright violet, betanaphthol to yield red-brown and hydroquinone to yield yellow-brown.[23]

Products designed for home use are not able to affect as dramatic a color change as those developed for professional salon use. Home-use dyes can only cover 35% gray hair and those with more gray hair will need to seek the expertise of a professional colorist. In Figures 4.13–4.20 the technique for professional salon hair dyeing is demonstrated with a demipermanent dye designed to cover and tone gray hair for 10–12 shampooings. Following this procedure, the dye is then rinsed and a conditioner is applied as previously discussed for the home-use hair dyes. This technique is basically for dyeing all of the hair shafts the same color. Currently fashionable techniques call for dyeing the hair several different colors to simulate the color variation present in natural undyed hair. One of the frequent complaints about dyed hair is the flat look

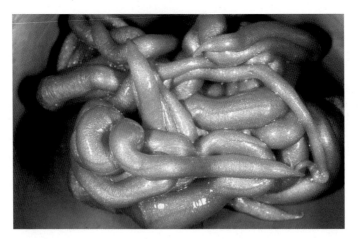

Figure 4.13
The dye is first squeezed from the tube into a bowl.

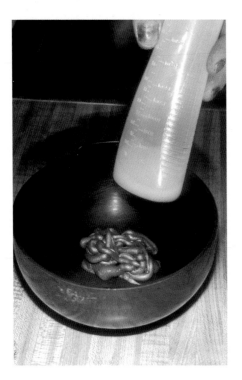

Figure 4.14
The hydrogen peroxide activator is
added.

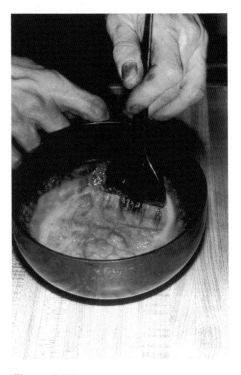

Figure 4.15
The completed dye mixture is stirred
to begin the chemical reaction.

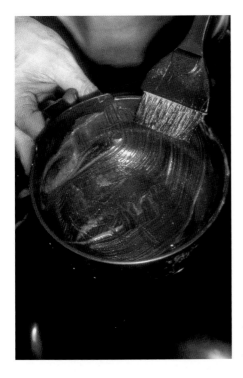

Figure 4.16
The activated dye is removed from the mixing bowl on a stiff brush for application to the hair.

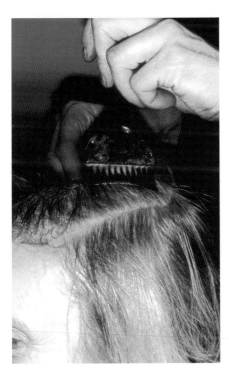

Figure 4.17
The hair is parted into quarter-inch sections and the hair is brushed with the dye.

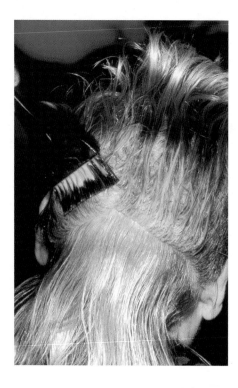

Figure 4.18
The dye is applied to the hair at the front of the head first, followed by the back of the head, and left in place for 25 minutes.

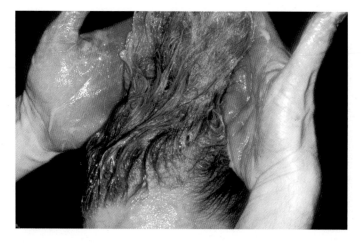

Figure 4.19
The dye is worked into the entire scalp including the ends of the hair shafts for the last 10 minutes.

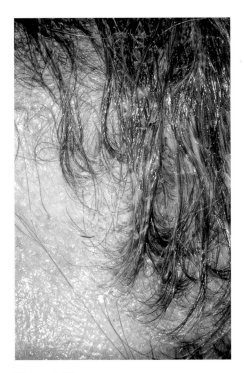

Figure 4.20
The appearance of the freshly applied dye on the hair shaft.

that it possesses. This is due to the absence of natural color variation, known as hair highlights. 'Highlighting' is a specialty dyeing technique designed to artificially create color variations in dyed hair, which is the next topic of discussion.

Specialty dyeing techniques

A relatively new trend in permanent hair dyeing is the technique of 'highlighting,' also known as 'hair foiling.' This technique involves the application of permanent hair dye to selected locks of hair that are then wrapped in the type of aluminum foil sheets used to cover oven-baked potatoes. The foil keeps the hair dye from touching surrounding hair and preferentially dyes only the intended locks. Hairdressers may foil one lock of hair red, another lock of hair light brown, and another lock of hair blond to create dramatic color variation. If large clumps of hair are dyed different colors, the effect looks quite artificial, however, if small clumps of hair are dyed different colors the variation creates a more cosmetically pleasing appearance. It is the natural variation in hair shaft color that gives natural hair some of its luster and shine, which can be created with foiling.

Foiling is popular among mature men and women. It is normal for the hair of the side burns and temple to gray before the top of the scalp in men and women. In order to minimize the amount of gray hair, while preserving some of the natural gray color, hair coloring artists are selectively dyeing the hair on the top of the head with minimal or no dye application to the temples. Sometimes blond highlights are added around the face to give the 'sun-kissed' look, which naturally results from UV-induced hair bleaching. These techniques of hair painting have become so artistic that many salons offer hair color services only and do not cut or style hair. A popular hair colorist can charge $200–$500 for this artistic type of hair blending.

The technique for hair foiling is illustrated in Figures 4.21–4.36 using a naturally red-headed woman with 25% gray hair who elects to undergo a highlighting procedure with three colors to yield light brown, red, and blond hair variations.

Highlighting using the foiling method can be accomplished using any dye color combinations desired. Individuals with brown hair can achieve blond highlights, as shown in Figure 4.37, or various shades of golden hair can be created, as shown in Figure 4.38.

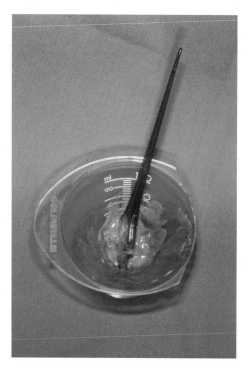

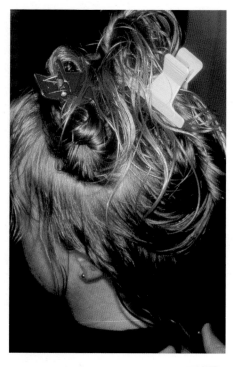

Figure 4.21
The brown permanent hair dye is mixed
using a black brush for identification.

Figure 4.22
The hair is pinned and sectioned prior
to dyeing.

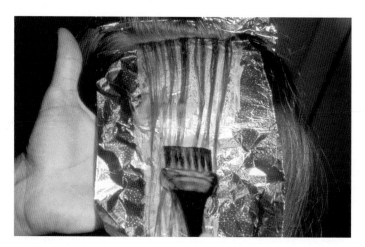

Figure 4.23
Selected sections are painted with the brown dye over a thin
foil.

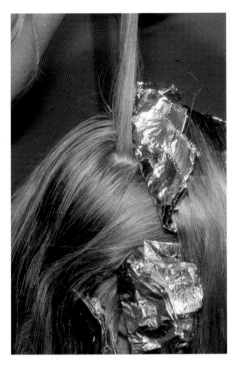

Figure 4.24
The foil is wrapped to create a pouch
that is placed on the top of the head.

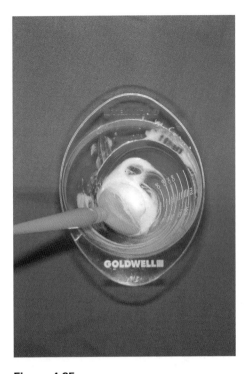

Figure 4.25
The blond permanent hair dye is mixed
using a gray brush for identification.

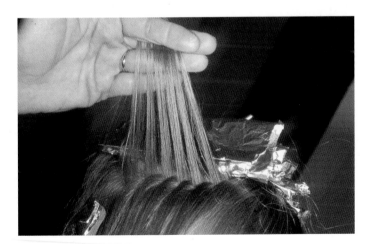

Figure 4.26
The hair sections to be dyed blond are selected by hand.

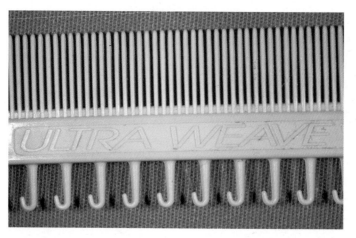

Figure 4.27
A special hook comb can also be used to select the strands
of hair for dyeing.

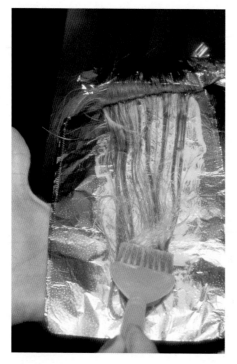

Figure 4.28
The selected hair sections are painted
with the blond dye.

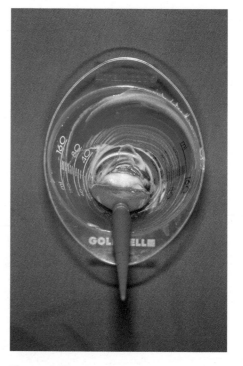

Figure 4.29
The red permanent hair dye is mixed
using a red brush for identification.

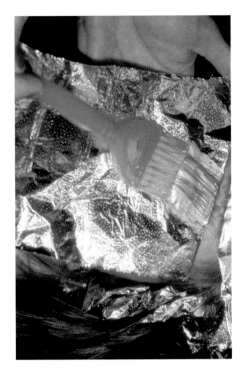

Figure 4.30
The red dye is applied to the selected hair
shafts and sealed in foil.

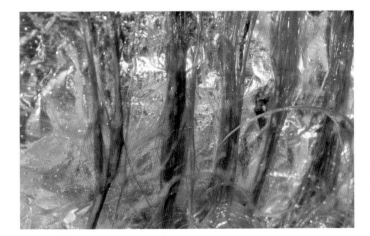

Figure 4.31
After the desired period of time,
usually 20–30 minutes, the hair is
removed from the foil wrap as shown
here with the dyed red strands.

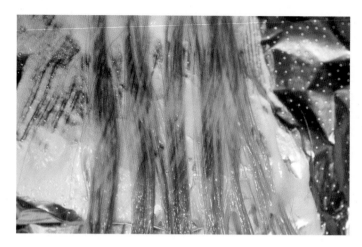

Figure 4.32
The appearance of the blond strands immediately after foil unwrapping.

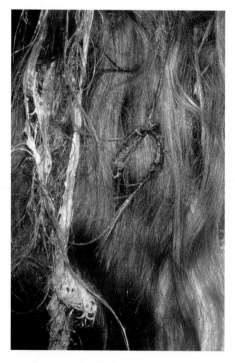

Figure 4.33
The multicolored strands of hair are apparent immediately after foil unwrapping.

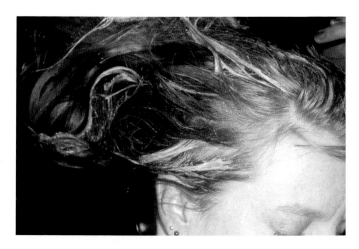

Figure 4.34
The hair is rinsed thoroughly to remove any remaining hair dye.

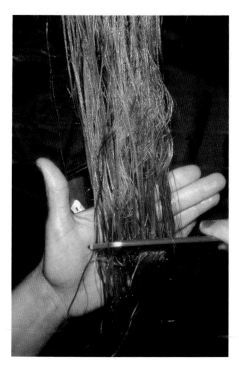

Figure 4.35
The hair is combed and dried.

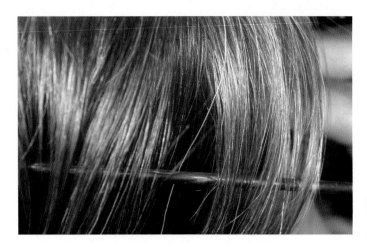

Figure 4.36
The final styled appearance of the dyed hair.

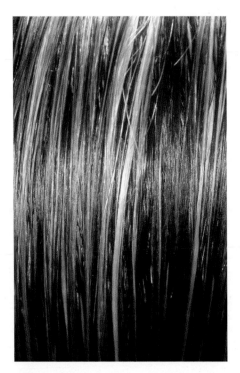

Figure 4.37
Brown hair with blond foiled highlights.

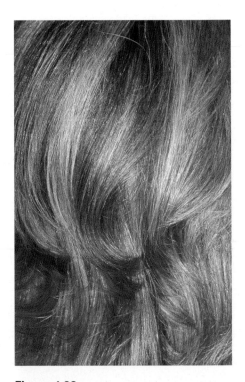

Figure 4.38
Brown hair foiled with numerous golden shades.

Minimizing hair damage

Permanent hair dyes are the most damaging to the hair because the dye alters the internal hair shaft structure, resulting in decreased tensile strength (Figure 4.39). Box 4.1 lists the key points to remember when advising patients regarding the use of permanent hair dyes.

HAIR COLOR LIGHTENING

Hair color can be lightened or 'bleached' with one-step or two-step processing. In one-step processing, the dyeing and lightening procedures are performed as one step, but the hair cannot be dramatically lightened. For example, a brunette could not be dyed to a golden blond color. One-step processing uses the same dyes as discussed previously, except the hydrogen peroxide used in the oxidation dyeing process is used to lighten the existing hair color, a

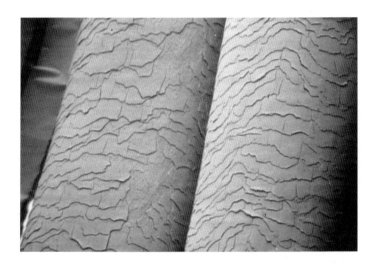

Figure 4.39
Permanently dyed hair irreversibly damaged due to cuticle loss.

Box 4.1 Minimizing hair dye damage

1. Do not attempt to lighten or darken hair by more than three shades.
2. Minimize the exposure of the hair to dye by prolonging the interval between dyeing sessions.
3. If possible, always dye hair darker not lighter. Bleaching is more damaging than dyeing.
4. If both permanent waving and permanent dyeing are to be performed, the hair should be permanently waved first and permanently dyed second.
5. Allow 10 days between permanent dyeing and permanent waving procedures.
6. Minimize shampooing to prolong the life of the hair dye.

phenomenon known as 'lift.' Permanent hair dyes designed to darken the hair must actually be carefully formulated to avoid lift. This inadvertent lightening due to the hydrogen peroxide required to initiate the oxidation/reduction reaction is used to create lighter hair color shades in the one-step process.

Two-step hair processing involves removing the natural hair pigments followed by dyeing to the desired lighter shade. This technique is used when patients wish to dye their hair much lighter than their natural color or if the hair contains more than 60% gray and darkening the hair color would be difficult. Removal of the natural hair pigments, a process known as hair bleaching, is achieved with an alkaline mixture of hydrogen peroxide and ammonia. This causes swelling of the hair shaft, allowing easier penetration of the dye, known as a toner.[25] The toner must be used since hair completely stripped of color has an undesirable grayish appearance. The toner can be selected either from the permanent or semi-permanent family of dyes.

Two-step bleaching is actually a complex chemical reaction involving melanin that occurs within the hair shaft. Melanin pigment has a unique chemical composition that is very resistant to reducing agents, but easily degraded by oxidizing agents. Thus, hair bleaching is an oxidative alkaline reaction. Hydrogen peroxide is the major oxidizer in the process, causing oxygen to be released from the hair keratin. The amount of hair lightening obtained is directly proportional to the amount of oxygen released from the hair shaft. In the hair dyeing industry, the quantity of oxygen released is expressed as 'volumes.' The volume of a hydrogen peroxide solution is the number of liters of oxygen released by a liter of the bleaching solution. For example, a 20 volume solution contains 6% hydrogen peroxide and a 30 volume solution contains 9% hydrogen peroxide.[26]

Hair bleaching products have been developed for both home and professional use. The home bleaching products generally contain 6% hydrogen peroxide and professional bleaching products may contain up to 9% hydrogen peroxide. It is felt that only a trained hair professional can safely apply the higher volumes of hydrogen peroxide. Hair bleach is applied to dry unwashed hair, since sebum minimizes scalp irritation. The bleaching oxidative alkaline reaction is initiated by mixing the hydrogen peroxide solution with an alkaline ammonia solution to obtain a pH of 9–11. The ammonia serves to speed the bleaching reaction, but must be used in the smallest amount possible to minimize excess keratin damage and scalp irritation. The reaction occurs most rapidly at the scalp due to the presence of body heat. For this reason, proper bleaching requires that the solution be applied at the hair ends first and then the roots to ensure an even color throughout the hair shaft. The bleaching solution is left on the hair for the desired amount of time and then removed with a low surfactant acidic pH shampoo. This reverses the hair shaft swelling induced by the high pH bleaching chemicals and minimizes hair damage. The newly bleached hair is then dried and styled as desired.

To achieve dramatic hair color lightening, the hair must be lightened to the desired color group and then dyed to the desired shade. There are seven basic levels of hair color from which the patient can select (Box 4.2). Each level must be traversed to reach the desired lighter hair color. A woman with black natural hair color would have to go through all seven stages of lightening to become a pale yellow blonde, whereas a woman with natural gold hair color would have to go through three stages of lightening to become a pale yellow blonde.

Understanding the levels of hair lightening is important, since it allows the physi-

Box 4.2 Levels of hair color

1. Black
2. Brown
3. Red
4. Red gold
5. Gold
6. Yellow
7. Pale yellow

Note: Hair colors are listed from darkest to lightest.

cian to predict how much hair damage must be sustained to achieve the desired lighter hair color. The more stages of lightening required to achieve the desired hair color, the stronger the bleaching agent that must be used and the more damaging the process is to the hair.[27] Often, such drastic hair lightening is desired that it cannot be achieved with hydrogen peroxide alone. In this case, a 'booster,' such as ammonium persulfate or potassium persulfate, may be added to the hydrogen peroxide and ammonia bleaching solution.[28] The eumelanin pigments in the hair are easily bleached by hydrogen peroxide, but the pheomelanins are somewhat resistant. This accounts for the need to use a booster when bleaching red hair.

Specialty bleaching techniques

There are a variety of popular bleaching techniques that involve lightening some, but not all, of the hairs on the scalp. These techniques are quite similar to the hair foiling procedures discussed previously. As a matter of fact, when the blond hair dye was applied to the selected scalp hairs of the subject in Figure 4.28, this was actually one-step hair bleaching. There are some currently fashionable patterns of hair bleaching that should be additionally discussed.

There are other methods of selectively bleaching selected groups of hairs in addition to foiling. One technique utilizes a tight fitting cap with holes that is placed over the head. The special hooked comb shown in Figure 4.27 is used to pull the entire hairs through the cap, which are then painted with the hair bleach along their entire length, a process known as 'frosting.' If only the tips of selected locks of hair are pulled through the cap and painted with bleach, the process is known as 'tipping.' If very large clumps of hair are pulled through the cap and bleached along their entire length, the process is known as 'streaking.' Fashion trends dictate the proportion of bleached to unbleached hairs in the scalp. These methods of selective hair bleaching are popular among brunette women who are graying to camouflage the presence of gray hairs.

Minimizing hair damage

Bleaching is extremely damaging to the hair shaft (Figure 4.40). Following the procedure there is a 2–3% weight loss from each individual shaft, resulting in decreased tensile strength and increased hair breakage. This is due to degradation of the amino acids tyrosine, threonine, and methionine combined with a loss of 15–25% of the hair disulfide bonds and 45% of the cystine bonds.[29] This weakening of the hair shaft is more pronounced in wet hair, thus bleached hair should be handled minimally until dry.[30] Bleached hair is also more porous due to loss of the cuticular scale and tends to absorb water, increasing its susceptibility to humidity changes. Decreased overlapping of the cuticular scale also leads to increased hair friction, which allows the hair to tangle more readily. In summary, hair that has been bleached is extremely porous and as a result is brittle, hard to untangle, and lacking in luster. Conditioners can do very little to

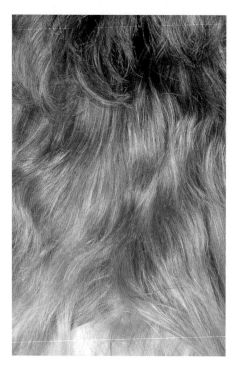

Figure 4.40
The appearance of damaged bleached hair.

improve the appearance of hair that has sustained such severe damage.

Most patients with bleached hair who are dissatisfied with the appearance and texture of their hair are best advised to cut the damaged portion of the hair shafts and await new growth. Unfortunately, once the hair has been bleached many shades lighter than the natural hair color, the proximal dark regrowth is cosmetically unattractive. Alternatives include changing to a shorter hairstyle, wearing a wig during the regrowth period, or using a semipermanent dye to blend the bleached and naturally colored areas of the hair shaft.

HAIR DYE REMOVAL

Occasionally, it becomes necessary to remove hair dye either due to a poor color result or the incompatibility of one dye with another chemical hair process. Removal of hair dye depends upon the type of coloring process used. As discussed previously, temporary hair dyes are removed with one shampooing while semipermanent hair dyes are removed in four to six shampooings. The amount of time for a dye to wash out is equal to the time required for the dye to color the hair shaft. For example, if it takes 20 minutes for a semipermanent dye to penetrate from the cuticle to the cortex, then it will also take 20 minutes for the dye to exit the hair shaft. Thus, if the hair is shampooed for 5 minutes, the dye will be removed in four shampooings for a total elapsed time of 20 minutes. Typically, hair dye removal is not a problem with temporary or semipermanent dyes and most patients are willing to wait while the undesirable color disappears.

Permanent hair dye removal is a much different matter, however. It is actually easier to bleach hair than to remove these unnatural pigments. Permanent dyes can be removed with either reducing agents or oxidants. High strength hydrogen peroxide, a strong oxidant, can be used but color lightening will occur. Sodium hydrosulfite or sodium formaldehyde sulfoxylate, which are strong reducing agents, can also be used. Permanent hair dye can be removed by dissolving 2–5% sodium hydrosulfite in water followed by an alkaline rinse.[27] Special salon removal products can also be used (Metalux, Clairol), but extreme hair damage results no matter what product is selected. If possible, it is recommended that other temporary or semipermanent dyes be used to tone the poorly colored hair until it can be trimmed.

Gradual hair dyes, also known as metallic dyes, may also require removal from the hair, since they are incompatible with permanent waving procedures. Gradual hair dyes should not be removed with peroxide as the hair can become darkened or discolored. Sulfonated castor oil with the addition of salicylic acid or chelating agents may be used.[31] Again, it is recommended that the dyed hair is trimmed away and replaced with new growth before attempting to remove the metallic dye.

HAIR COLORING IN AFRICAN-AMERICANS

Hair coloring techniques available to the African-American patient are the same as those discussed for the Caucasian patient. Many dyes in temporary, semipermanent, demipermanent, and permanent formulations are available for darkening the hair color of the African-American patient. This can be done for fashion reasons or to cover gray hair. Darkening the hair color is not as damaging as lightening the hair color, but may result in excessive hair breakage, if permanent hair coloring is combined with chemical straightening. However, if bleaching or lightening of the hair is desired, high volume peroxide is required, which can be extremely damaging to the hair shaft. If African-American hair is lightened, it usually bleaches to a red color as the pheomelanins are not easily removed. If hair bleaching is combined with hair straightening, the hair is so severely damaged that it cannot withstand the trauma of routine grooming. The hair breaks at its exit point from the scalp, leaving the patient with thin ungroomable hair.

HAIR DYE ALLERGY

The allergic potential of hair dyes due to the presence of paraphenylenediamine is well known to the dermatologist. Paraphenylenediamine is found on all standardized patch test trays and also on the TRUE test patches. The allergy is characterized by scalp pruritus and erythema when mild and facial edema and eye swelling when severe (Figure 4.41). All hair dye product manufacturers recommend applying a small amount

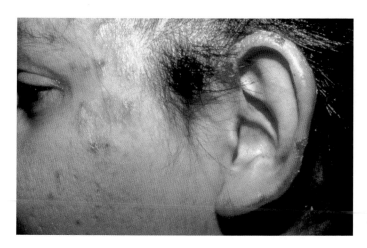

Figure 4.41
A mild hair dye reaction to paraphenylenediamine.

of the dye to a localized area of hair prior to dyeing the entire scalp as a test to rule out the possibility of allergic contact dermatitis. Hair dye inserts recommend that this test be repeated prior to each dye contact.

Gradual and temporary hair dyes represent minimal risk for irritant and allergic contact dermatitis, since they contain no paraphenylenediamine. Semipermanent dyes are a cause of allergic contact dermatitis since they may contain 'para' dyes (diamines, aminophenols and phenols) or dyes that cross-react with the 'para' dyes. Permanent hair dyes contain the highest concentration of paraphenylenediamine (PPD),[32] with an estimated incidence of allergic contact dermatitis of 1 in every 50,000 applications.[33] However, patch testing may overestimate the incidence of reactions to PPD-containing hair dyes. This is due to the limited contact time during dyeing and the less than 3% concentration of PPD present in most permanent dyes. Furthermore, PPD rapidly combines with the hair dye oxidizing agent to create a new chemical moiety.[34]

It is possible that a patient may be allergic to one 'para' dye and not another. In special cases, it may be worthwhile to test to each individual dye rather than using the standard patch test tray PPD formulation. The individual dyes that can be tested and their formulations for patch testing are listed in Box 4.3.[35]

Once the hair has been semipermanently or permanently dyed, it is no longer allergenic,[36] but all excess dye must be removed with a final acidic shampoo, known as a neutralizing rinse. Sometimes patients with a severe para-phenylenediamine allergy, who have previously used home dyeing preparations, develop swelling and bullae formation immediately upon application of the dye product. In their haste to come to the dermatologist's office, they may neglect to remove all of the excess dye. Schueller recommends a chloride peroxide rinse to neutralize the excess dye, which is formulated as follows:[37]

- Sodium chloride, 150 g
- Hydrogen peroxide (20 volume), 50 ml
- Water, q.s. 1000 ml

This preparation can be mixed by the pharmacist and applied to the patient's hair to remove any remaining allergen. It is not necessary for the patient to cut his or her hair, but further hair dyeing should be avoided.

Hair bleaching has also been reported to cause hair breakage, skin irritation, allergic sensitization, and scarring alopecia.[38] Cutaneous and respiratory allergic reactions have been reported to ammonium persulfate, mentioned previously as a booster in the hair bleaching process.[39] Reported reactions include: allergic contact dermatitis, irri-

---

Box 4.3 Hair dye allergy extended patch testing ingredients

- Para-phenylenediamine, 1% in petrolatum
- Para-toluylenediamine, 1% in petrolatum
- Ortho-nitroparaphenylenediamine, 1% in petrolatum
- Meta-toluylenediamine, 1% in petrolatum
- Resorcinol, 2% in petrolatum
- Meta-aminophenol, 2% in petrolatum
- Hydroquinone, 1% in petrolatum

tant contact dermatitis, localized edema, generalized urticaria, rhinitis, asthma, and syncope.[40,41] Some of the reactions are thought to be truly allergic while others appear to be due to nonimmunologic histamine release.[42] Patch testing may be performed with a 2–5% aqueous solution of ammonium persulfate to obtain further patient information.[43]

SAFETY ISSUES

Hair coloring products are generally regarded as safe products with low risk of mutagenicity and oncogenicity.[44–46] There has been some concern recently in the popular press regarding the safe use of hair dyes in pregnant women. Research conducted within the hair care industry has demonstrated that the skin penetration is minimal and limited to 0.02–0.2% of the quantity of dye applied to the head.[47,48] Furthermore, a prospective study of permanent hair dye use found no increase in hematopoietic cancers.[49] Carcinogenicity was a concern due to the presence of aromatic amines in hair dyes. These aromatic amines were found to cause tumors in rodents fed the maximum tolerated dose at the National Cancer Institute (NCI).

THE FUTURE

The next frontier in hair color will be the prevention of gray hair through melanocyte stimulating factors and the natural alteration of hair color through the use of melanin modulators. This technology is currently at the petri dish stage. Ongoing cooperative research between my laboratory and others has been slowed by the need to develop sta-

ble melanocyte cultures from the hair bulb to test chemicals designed to alter the production of eumelanin and pheomelanin. The fragility of hair melanocyte cultures has slowed the research, but several commonly encountered safe substances show great promise. Other research is focusing on techniques of removing toxic oxidative melanin byproducts from the follicular melanocytes, which theoretically may allow remelanization to occur.[50] Even others are evaluating the use of melanin itself as a more natural appearing hair dye.[51,52] For the time being, however, we shall have to be content with dyes that create color changes synthetically.

REFERENCES

1. Casperson S. Men's hair coloring: a review of current technology. *Cosmet Toilet* 1994;**109**: 83–7.
2. Corbett J. Hair coloring processes. *Cosmet Toilet* 1991;**106**:53–7.
3. Menkart J, Wolfram LJ, Mao I. Caucasian hair, negro hair, and wool; similarities and differences. *J Soc Cosmet Chem* 1966; **17**:769–89.
4. Arakindakshan MI, Persad S, Haberman HF, Kurian CJ. A comparative study of the physical and chemical properties of melanins isolated from human black and red hair. *J Invest Dermatol* 1983;**80**:202–6.
5. Brown KC, Prota G. Melanins: hair dyes for the future. *Cosmet Toilet* 1994;**109**: 59–64.
6. Cesarini JP. Hair melanin and hair colour. In: Orfanos CE, Happle R, eds. *Hair and hair diseases*. Berlin: Springer-Verlag, 1990:166–97.
7. Vardy DA, Marcus B, Gilead L *et al*. A look at gray hair. *J Geriatric Dermatol* 1993;**1**:22–7.
8. Pohl S. The chemistry of hair dyes. *Cosmet Toilet* 1988;**103**:1988:57–66.
9. Spoor HJ. Part II: Metals. *Cutis* 1977; **19**:37–40.
10. O'Donoghue MN. Hair cosmetics. *Dermatol Clin* 1987;**5**:619–25.

11. Casperson S. Men's hair coloring. *Cosmet Toilet* 1994:**109**:83–7.

12. Spoor HJ. Hair dyes: temporary colorings. *Cutis* 1976;**18**:341–4.

13. Corbett JF. Hair coloring. *Clin Dermatol* 1988;**6**:93–101.

14. Wilkinson JB, Moore RJ. *Harry's cosmeticology*, 7th edn. New York: Chemical Publishing, 1982:526–8.

15. Corbett JF. Hair dyes. In: *The chemistry of synthetic dyes*, Vol 5. New York: Academic Press, 1971:475–534.

16. Spoor HJ. Semi-permanent hair color. *Cutis* 1976;**18**:506–8.

17. Corbett JF. Hair coloring processes. *Cosmet Toilet* 1991;**106**:53.

18. Robbin CR. *Chemical and physical behavior of human hair*, 2nd edn. New York: Springer-Verlag, 1988:185–8.

19. Zviak C. Hair coloring, nonoxidation coloring. In: Zviak C, ed. *The science of hair care*. New York: Marcel Dekker, 1986:235–61.

20. Tucker HH: Formulation of oxidation hair dyes. *Am J Perfum Cosmet* 1968;**83**:69.

21. Corbett JF, Menkart J. Hair coloring. *Cutis* 1973;**12**:190.

22. Zviak C. Oxidation coloring. In: Zviak C, ed. *The science of hair care*. New York: Marcel Dekker, 1986:263–86.

23. Spoor HJ. Permanent hair colorants: oxidation dyes. Part II Colorist's art. *Cutis* 1977;**19**:578–88.

24. Corbett JF. Chemistry of hair colorant processes – science as an aid to formulation and development. *J Soc Cosmet Chem* 1984:**35**:297–310.

25. Spoor HJ. Hair coloring – a resume. *Cutis* 1977;**20**:311–13.

26. Kass GS. Hair coloring products. In: deNavarre MG, ed. *The chemistry and manufacture of cosmetics*, Vol IV, 2nd edn. Wheaton IL: Allured Publishing Corporation, 1988:841–920.

27. Zviak C. Hair bleaching. In: Zviak C, ed. *The science of hair care*. New York: Marcel Dekker, 1986:213–33.

28. Corbett JF. Hair coloring processes. *Cosmet Toilet* 1991;**106**:53–7.

29. Robbins C, Kelly. Amino acid analysis of cosmetically altered hair. *J Soc Cosmet Chem* 1969;**20**:555–64.

30. Robbins CR. Physicial properties and cosmetic behavior of hair. In: *Chemical and physical behavior of human hair*, 2nd edn. New York: Springer-Verlag, 1988:225–8.

31. Wall, FE. Bleaches, hair colorings, and dye removers. In: Balsam MS, Gershon SD, Rieger MM, Sagarin E, Strianse SJ, eds. *Cosmetics science and technology*, Vol 2, 2nd edn. New York: Wiley-Interscience, 1972: 279–343.

32. Goldberg BJ, Herman FF, Hirata I. Systemic anaphylaxis due to an oxidation product of p-phenylenediamine in a hair dye. *Ann Allergy* 1987;**58**:205–8.

33. Rostenberg A, Kass GS. *Hair coloring*. AMA Committee of Cutaneous Health and Cosmetics, 1969.

34. Corbett JF. p-benzoquinonediimine – a vital intermediate in oxidative hair dyeing. *J Soc Cosmetic Chemists* 1969;**20**:253.

35. DeGroot AC, Weyland JW, Nater JP. *Unwanted effects of cosmetics and drugs used in dermatology*, Amsterdam: Elsevier, 1994:481–2.

36. Reiss F, Fisher AA. Is hair dyed with para-phenylenediamine allergenic? *Arch Dermatol* 1974;**109**:221–2.

37. Calnan C. Adverse reactions to hair products. In: Zviak C, ed. *The science of hair care*. New York: Marcel Dekker, 1986:409–23.

38. Bergfeld WF. Orfanos CE, Montagna E, Stuttgen G, eds. *Hair research*. Berlin: Springer-Verlag, 1981:534–7.

39. Fisher AA, Dooms-Goossens A. Persulfate hair bleach reactions. *Arch Dermatol* 1976;**112**:1407.

40. Brubaker MM. Urticarial reaction to ammonium persulfate. *Arch Dermatol* 1972;**106**:413–14.

41. Blainey AD, Ollier S, Cundell D, Smith RE, Davies RJ. Occupational asthma in a hairdressing salon. *Thorax* 1986;**41**:42–50.

42. Calnan CD, Shuster S. Reactions to ammonium persulfate. *Arch Dermatol* 1963;**88**:812–15.

43. Fisher AA, Dooms-Goossens A. Persulfate hair bleach reactions. *Arch Dermatol* 1976;**112**:1407–9,

44. Marcoux D, Riboulet-Delmas G. Efficacy and safety of hair-coloring agents. *Am J Contact Dermatitis* 1994;**5**:123–9.

45. Morikawa F, Fujii S, Tejima M, Sugiyama H, Uzuak M. Safety evaluation of hair cosmetics. In: Kobori T, Montagna W, eds. *Biology and disease of the hair*. Baltimore: University Park Press, 1975;641–57.

46. Corbett JF. Hair dye toxicity. In: Orfanos CE, Montagna W, Stuttgen G, eds. *Hair research*. Springer-Verlag, 1981:529–35.

47. Kalopissis G. Toxicology and hair dyes. In: Zviak C, ed. *The science of hair care*. New York: Marcel Dekker, 1986:287–308.

48. Beck H, Bracher M, Faller C, Hofer H. Comparison of in vitro and in vivo skin permeation of hair dyes. *Cosmet Toilet* 1993; **108**:76–83.

49. Grodstein F, Hennekens CH, Colditz GA, Hunter DJ, Stampfer MJ. A prospective study of permanent hair dye use and hematopoietic cancer. *J Natl Cancer Inst* 1994;**86**: 1466–70.

50. Tobin D. Prevention and reversal of hair graying: a possibility? *Cosmet Toilet* 1998;**113**: 89–98.

51. Brown K, Prota G. Melanins: hair dyes for the future. *Cosmet Toilet* 1994;**109**:59–64.

52. Brown K, Marlowe E, Prota G, Wenke G. A novel natural-based hair coloring process. *J Soc Cosmet Chem* 1997;**48**:133–40.

5   Permanent hair curling

The idea of making straight hair permanently curly is not new. The first permanent hair waving procedure was developed by Nessler in 1906 and consisted of a borax paste applied to the hair followed by the use of external heat in the form of electrically heated hollow iron tubes. Later it was refined by combining the borax paste with heat generated by a chemical heating pad attached to the curling rods with a clamp. Temperatures reached about 115 degrees Centigrade and heating continued for 10–15 minutes.[1] Unfortunately, this procedure was very damaging to the hair. The idea of the cold permanent wave was introduced in the 1930s and immediately replaced the heat wave method. The cold waving solution contained ammonium thioglycolate and free ammonia at a controlled pH. This technique was patented in the United States by McDonough on June 16, 1941. Interestingly enough, this cold wave solution, with slight variations, is still popular today for both salon and home use. It is estimated that more than 65 million permanent waves are sold in salons and 45 million home waves are performed on an annual basis in the United States.[2]

CHEMISTRY

The chemistry of the permanent waving process is based on the 16% cystine incorporated into disulfide linkages between polypeptide chains in the hair keratin filament. These disulfide linkages are responsible for hair elasticity and can be reformed to change the configuration of the hair shaft. Permanent waving utilizes three processes: chemical softening, rearranging, and fixing of the disulfide bonds.[3] The basic chemistry involves the reduction of the disulfide hair shaft bonds with mercaptans and can be chemically characterized as shown in Box 5.1.[4,5]

Once the hair has undergone the permanent waving process, the hair must be evaluated for degree of curl versus degree of hair shaft damage.[6] The most common industry evaluation techniques are known as the deficiency in tightness value, the curl length, and the 20% index.[7] The deficiency in tightness (DIT) value is a measure of the tightness of the curl and is shown in Box 5.2. The higher the DIT value, the greater the effectiveness of the curling solution and the tighter the curl.

Box 5.1 Permanent hair waving chemistry

1. Penetration of the thiol compound into the hair shaft.
2. Cleavage of the hair keratin disulfide bond (kSSk) to produce a cysteine residue (kSH) and the mixed disulfide of the thiol compound with the hair keratin (kSSR).

$$kSSk + RSH \rightarrow kSH + kSSR$$

3. Reaction with another thiol molecule to produce a second cysteine residue and the symmetrical disulfide of the thiol waving agent (RSSR).

$$kSSR + RSH \rightarrow kSH + RSSR$$

4. Rearrangement of the hair protein structure to relieve internal stress determined by curler size and hair wrapping tension.
5. Application of an oxidizing agent to reform the disulfide cross-links.

$$kSH + HSk \xrightarrow{oxidizing\ agent} kSSk + water$$

Box 5.2 Deficiency in tightness value determination

DIT = diameter of curl (mm) − diameter of rod (mm)/diameter of the rod (mm) × 100

The curl length is an evaluation of the spring of the curl. The optimum curl is bouncy and springy, moving freely with motion of the body. The curl length is evaluated by suspending a fresh curl and observing the spring of the formed coil. The degree of laxity is proportional to the degree of hair shaft damage. Thus, longer curls are indicative of greater hair shaft damage.

Lastly, the 20% index is used to evaluate the strength of the permanently waved hair. The 20% index is determined by stretching freshly permed hair with a uniformly increasing load. The ratio of the load required after perming to the load required prior to perming to stretch a wet strand of 12 hairs to 20% of their original length is known as the 20% index. The higher the index, the lower the reduction in hair strength due to the cold wave procedure. Hair that has a low 20% index will break readily with minimal trauma, such as combing.

Hair cosmetic chemists use these criteria to assess the effect of the permanent waving chemicals on the hair shaft. Factors that must be considered when evaluating a permanent wave result are listed in Box 5.3.[8] An optimal permanent wave product must produce the best curl with the least amount of hair damage.[9]

APPLICATION TECHNIQUE

Cold permanent waves can be administered at home or in a salon, but involve the same application technique.[10] A permanent wave

---

Box 5.3 Factors affecting permanent wave efficacy

1. Processing time – longer processing time increases hair curl
2. Processing temperature – higher temperature increases hair curl
3. Concentration of reducing agent – higher reducing agent concentration increases hair curl
4. Ratio of lotion to hair quantity – larger quantity of waving lotion increases hair curl
5. Lotion penetration – increased waving lotion penetration increases hair curl
6. pH – higher pH increases hair curl
7. Condition of hair – good quality hair increases hair curl

---

usually can be completed in about 90 minutes depending on the length of the hair. It is an involved process of chemically and mechanically reforming the hair and is discussed step-by-step to help the physician understand how originally straight hair is transformed into curly hair.

The standard permanent waving procedure involves initial shampooing of the hair to remove dirt and sebum. This wetting process with water is the first step in preparing the hair for chemical treatment, since the water enters the hair's hydrogen bonds and allows increased flexibility. The hair is then sectioned into 30–50 areas (Figure 5.1), depending on the length and thickness of the hair, and wound on mandrels or rods with holes to allow the permanent waving solution to contact all surfaces of the hair shaft (Figure 5.2). The size of the rod determines the diameter of the curl, with smaller rods producing tighter curls and larger rods producing looser curls (Figure 5.3). The hair must be wound on the curling rod with sufficient tension to provide the stress required for bond breaking. If too much tension is applied, the hair can be stretched beyond its elastic range, transforming it into a brittle substance that will fracture easily.

Prior to wrapping the hair around the rods, the ends of the hair are wrapped in a thin sheet of tissue paper. The tissue paper squares are about 5 × 5 cm and are known as 'end papers' (Figure 5.4). End papers are applied to the distal hair shafts to prevent irregular wrapping of the ends around the rod (Figure 5.5). Failure to use end papers can result in a frizzy appearance of the distal hair shaft (Figure 5.6). The hair is then wrapped around the mandrel and secured

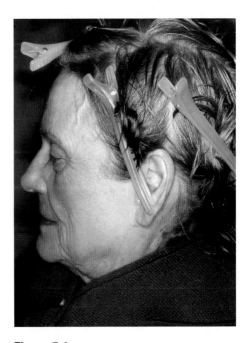

Figure 5.1
Hair sectioning for permanent wave.

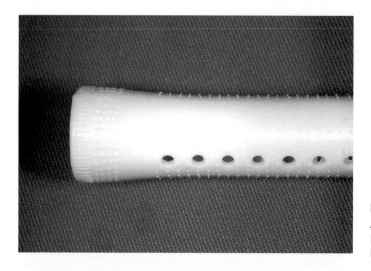

Figure 5.2
A curling rod containing holes for permanent waving lotion penetration.

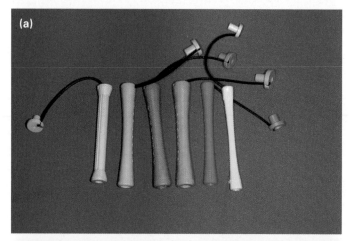

Figure 5.3
(a) A variety of smaller curling rods producing tight pin curls.

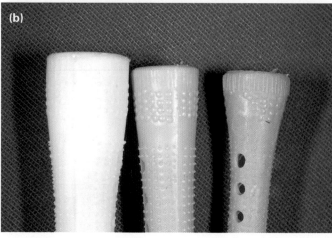

(b) A variety of larger curling rods producing larger body wave curls.

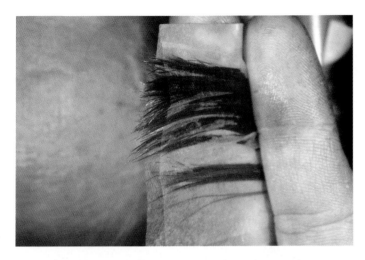

Figure 5.4
An end paper is demonstrated.

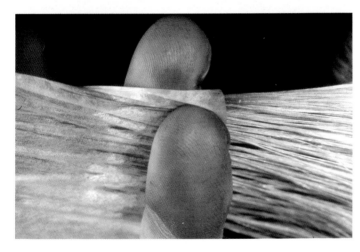

Figure 5.5
The hair must be evenly smooth over the end paper.

with a rubber band that is attached to an end cap on the end of the mandrel (Figure 5.7). It is important that the appropriate amount of tension is applied to the hair as it is wrapped around the mandrel. Tension is required to encourage the bond breaking process, but too little tension will result in poor curls while too much tension will result in damaged, brittle hair (Figure 5.8).

The hair is generally wrapped around the curling rods beginning at the back of the scalp (Figure 5.9). The beautician will continue to section and wrap the hair until a row of curlers has been placed over the middle of the scalp. The hair is always wrapped up from the neck forward to create the proper curl direction (Figure 5.10). The sides of the hair will then be wrapped down around mandrels until all of the hair has been placed on the mandrels. It is important to wrap the hair down on the sides to create the proper curl direction. Lastly, the beautician will check the tension on the rods and pull the attachment rubber bands down to the lower part of the curler. An absorbant piece of cotton is placed around the curlers to

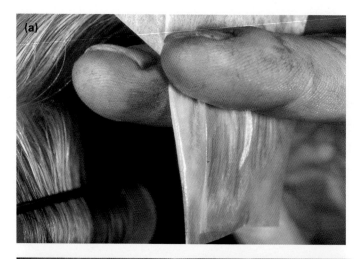

Figure 5.6
(a) The hair is completely wrapped in
the end paper.

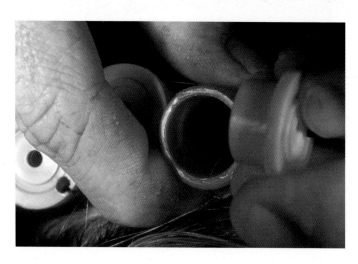

(b) The ends in the paper evenly
placed around the curling mandrel.

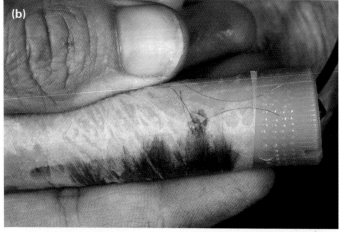

Figure 5.7
The end cap is inserted into the
curling mandrel.

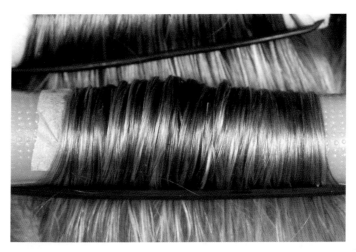

Figure 5.8
The hair is wrapped evenly around the curling mandrels
with the proper tension.

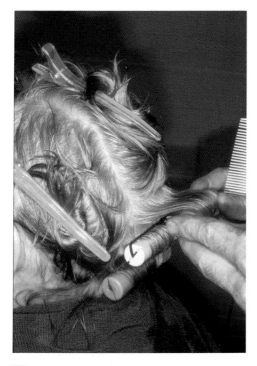

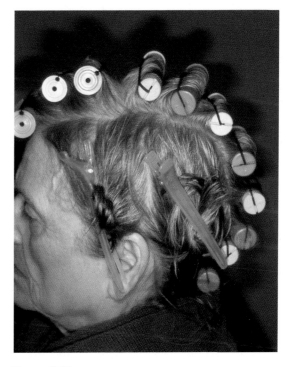

Figure 5.9
The hair is wrapped first at the nape of
the neck.

Figure 5.10
The mandrels have been placed over the middle
of the scalp with the hair rolled forward.

prevent the irritating waving lotion from contacting the scalp and the skin around the hairline (Figure 5.11).

After the hair has been completely wrapped on the curling rods, the waving lotion and the activator are mixed (Figure 5.12). The activated waving lotion is applied and left in contact with the hair for 5–20 minutes, depending on the condition of the hair (Figure 5.13). The reducing action of the waving lotion is said to 'soften' the hair and contains a disulfide bond-breaking agent, such as ammonium or calcium thioglycolate, and an antioxidant, such as sodium hydrosulfite, to prevent the lotion from reacting with air before it reaches the hair (Figure 5.14). Table 5.1 lists the basic ingredients in a waving lotion and their intended function. Other minor ingredients, such as

sequestering agents like tetrasodium EDTA, are added to prevent trace metals such as iron in tap water from reacting with the thioglycolate lotion. Minor ingredients such as pH adjusters, conditioners, and surfactants to remove the remaining sebum from the hair may be added.

Once the hair has been thoroughly saturated with the waving lotion, the hair is placed under a plastic shower cap (Figure 5.15). The cap traps the heat of the body, which is used to increase the activity of the permanent wave solution. The cap also traps the smell of sulfur, which is very characteristic in a salon where permanent waving is being performed. The sulfur smell, which resembles rotten eggs, is produced as sulfur escapes from the hair when the disulfide bonds are broken.

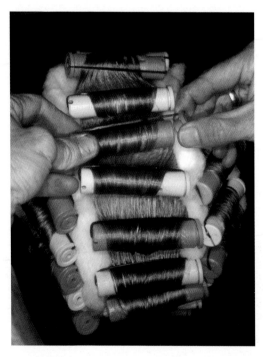

Figure 5.11
The rubber bands are adjusted and a cotton wick is placed around the curlers.

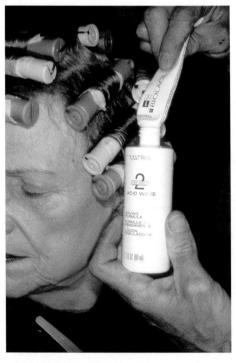

Figure 5.12
The waving lotion is activated.

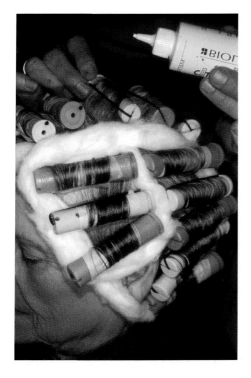

Figure 5.13
The activated waving lotion is applied to each curler.

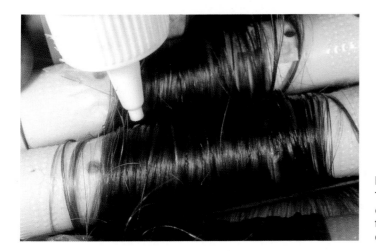

Figure 5.14
The waving lotion must be applied over the holes in the mandrel to thoroughly saturate the hair on the other side of the rod.

Table 5.1 Permanent waving lotion ingredients

Ingredient	Chemical examples	Function
Reducing agent	Thioglycolic acid thiolactic acid, glycerol monothioglycolate, sodium sulfite	Break disulfide bonds
Alkaline agent	Ammonium hydroxide, triethanolamine	Adjust pH
Chelating agent	Tetrasodium EDTA	Remove trace metals
Wetting agent	Fatty alcohols, sodium lauryl sulfate, disodium laureth sulfosuccinate, sodium laureth sulfate, cocoamphodiacetate	Improve hair saturation with waving lotion
Antioxidant	Tocopherol, tocopherol acetate	Preservative
Buffer	Ammonium carbonate	Adjust pH
Conditioner	Proteins, humectants, quaternium compounds	Protect hair during waving process
Opacifier	Polyacrylates, polystyrene latex	Opacify waving lotion

Adapted from Lee et al.[1]

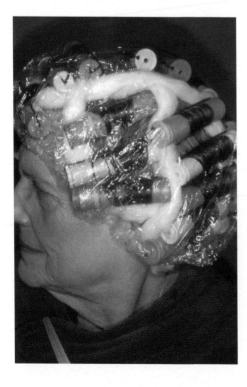

Figure 5.15
A plastic shower cap is placed over the head after the waving lotion has been applied.

The processing time for the permanent wave depends on the thickness and condition of the hair. Coarse hair requires a longer processing time than fine hair due to the longer time required for the waving lotion to penetrate a thicker diameter hair. If the hair has been previously chemically processed and the cuticle has been disrupted, the processing time is shorter. For example, undyed hair requires a longer processing time than permanently dyed or bleached hair. In order to avoid over- or under-processing the hair, a 'test curl' is checked to determine if the desired amount of curl has been obtained (Figure 5.16). The test curl is typically placed at the nape of the neck where the hair is the most resistant to permanent waving. This insures that an adequate amount of curl has been achieved over the entire scalp. A successful test curl has been achieved when the hair retains a 'C' shape when the curler is removed. If the hair is not in a 'C' shape, the permanent wave solution must be left in the hair longer to allow more bond-breaking to occur.

Once the desired amount of curl has been achieved, the hair disulfide bonds are reformed with the hair in the new curled conformation around the curling rods. This process is known as neutralization, fixation or 'hardening' (Figure 5.17). The neutralization procedure, chemically characterized as an oxidation step, involves two steps. First, two-thirds of the neutralizer are applied to

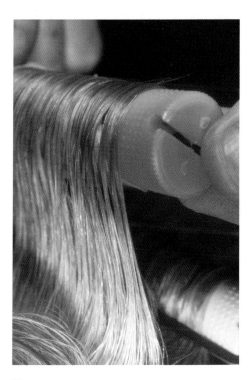

Figure 5.16
Assessment of a test curl to determine if the permanent wave is complete.

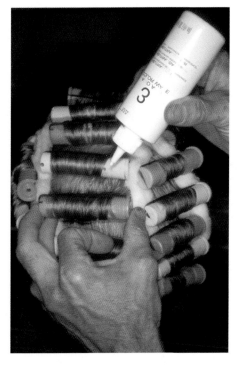

Figure 5.17
The hair is saturated with the neutralizer while on the curling rods.

thoroughly saturate the hair with the rods in place and allowed to set for 5 minutes. The rods are then removed and the remaining one-third of the neutralizer is applied for an additional 5 minutes (Figure 5.18). The hair is then carefully rinsed.

The neutralizer functions to reform the broken disulfide bonds and restores the hair to its original condition. Two methods are available, self-neutralization and chemical neutralization, relying on oxidation reaction. Self-neutralization allows air to oxidize the permanent wave, but this requires 6–24 hours. During this time, the hair must be left on the permanent wave rods. This method is rarely used. Chemical neutralization is more popular, due to its speed, and relies upon the use of an oxidizing agent. The oxidizing agent is usually 2% hydrogen peroxide adjusted to an acidic pH. Bromates may also be used, but are more expensive. The ingredients found in a chemical neutralizer and their function are summarized in Table 5.2.[11]

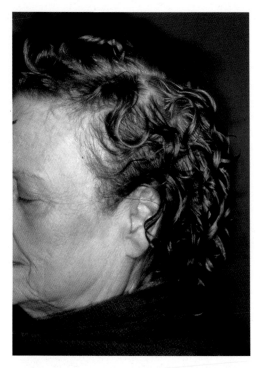

Figure 5.18
Appearance of the hair after removal of the curling rods.

Table 5.2 Permanent wave neutralizer ingredients

Ingredient	Chemical example	Function
Oxidizing agent	Hydrogen peroxide, sodium bromate	Reform broken disulfide bonds
Acid buffer	Citric acid, acetic acid, lactic acid	Maintain acidic pH
Stabilizer	Sodium stannate	Prevent hydrogen peroxide breakdown
Wetting agent	Fatty alcohols	Improve hair saturation with neutralizer
Conditioner	Proteins, humectants, quaternium compounds	Improve hair feel
Opacifier	Polyacrylates, polystyrene latex	Make neutralizer opaque

Adapted from Lee *et al*.[1]

The newly curled hair is now conditioned to prevent additional damage to the fragile hair shafts (Figure 5.19). The hair is then ready for drying and styling (Figure 5.20). Most companies recommend avoiding shampooing or manipulating the hair for 1–2 days after the cold wave procedure to insure long-lasting curls.

A permanent wave is designed to last 3–4 months. Curl relaxation occurs with time as the hair returns to its original conformation. Hairdressers generally will therefore select a curl tighter than the patient desires with this fact in mind (Figure 5.21). Most of the curl relaxation occurs within the first 2 weeks after processing, a fact that is reassuring to the patient who has had an undesirable result (Figure 5.22). Curl relaxation can be increased slightly by frequent shampooing, beginning immediately after the permanent waving procedure. Some strong detergent shampoos, such as those recommended for seborrheic dermatitis, cause rapid curl relaxation.

The final appearance of a permanent wave is determined by the size of the mandrels around which the hair was wrapped. Very tight curls, such as pin curls, are achieved by wrapping the hair around small curling rods (Figure 5.23). Pins curls are popular among mature women wishing to use the tight curl to add body and create the illusion of fullness with thinning hair. Conversely, loose waves, such as body waves, are achieved by wrapping the hair around large curling rods (Figure 5.24). Body waves are used to create wavy rather than curly hair.

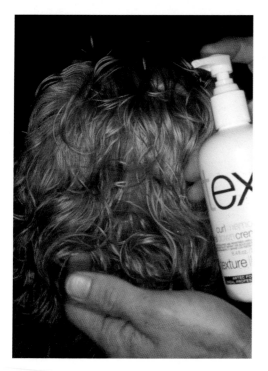

Figure 5.19
A styling conditioner is applied to the newly curled hair.

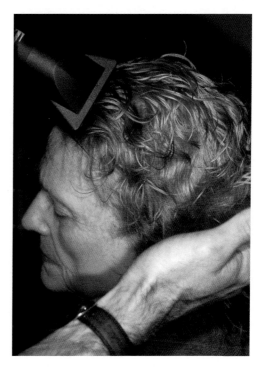

Figure 5.20
Hair drying following a permanent wave.

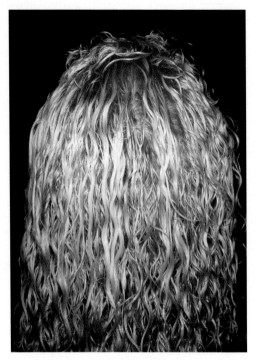

Figure 5.21
A tight curl.

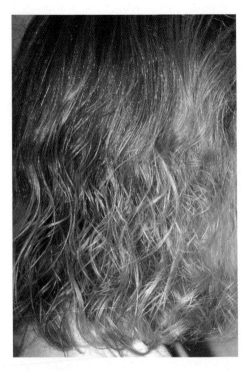

Figure 5.22
Relaxation of the curl.

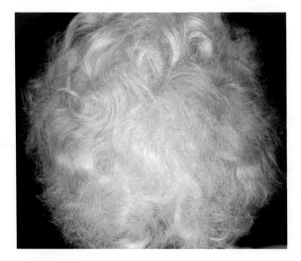

Figure 5.23
The appearance of pin curls created with a
permanent wave.

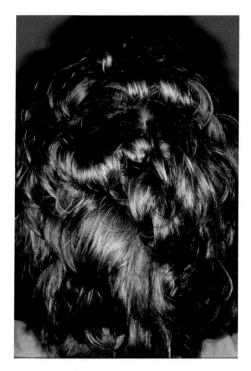

Figure 5.24
The appearance of a body wave.

TYPES OF PERMANENT WAVES

There are several types of permanent waves depending on the tightness of the wave and the chemistry of the solution employed. If the hair is wound on very small curling rods, the curls will be very tight, but if the hair is wound on larger rods, the curls will be loose. Tight curls are sometimes called pin curls (Figure 5.23), while loose curls are called a body wave (Figure 5.24). The diameter of the curl is a function of the curling rod and not the permanent waving solution. The rest of this discussion will focus on the various types of permanent wave solutions based on their unique chemistry.

The differences between the various types of permanent waves are due to the unique attributes of the waving lotions. Waving lotion consists primarily of a reducing agent in an aqueous solution with an adjusted pH.[11] The most popular reducing agents are the thioglycolates, glycerol thioglycolates, and sulfites. On the basis of waving lotion type, permanent waves can be classified into the groups listed in Table 5.3.[4,12]

Alkaline permanent waves

Alkaline permanent waves utilize ammonium thioglycolate or ethanolamine thioglycolate as the active reducing agent in the waving lotion. The pH of the waving lotion is adjusted to 9–10 since the thioglycolates are not effective at an acidic pH. Alkaline permanent waves produce tight, long-lasting curls very rapidly. The amount of time required to produce the curl is known as the 'processing time.' Thus, alkaline permanent waves have a short processing time. They are not a popular wave, however, since the hair is left inelastic and harsh. The alkalinity of the permanent wave produces hair shaft swelling, which irreversibly damages the cuticle. This can be problematic in individuals with color-treated hair, especially bleached hair. To minimize hair damage, the concentration of the alkaline thioglycolate waving lotion is adjusted from 7% for natural hair to 1% for bleached hair.

Buffered alkaline permanent waves

The high pH of the alkaline permanent wave can be reduced to minimize unnecessary hair damage. This has led to the development of the buffered alkaline permanent wave. In order to decrease hair swelling encountered from high pH alkaline permanent waves, a buffering agent, such as

Table 5.3 Types of permanent waves

Type of permanent wave	Chemistry	pH	Advantages	Disadvantages
Alkaline	Ammonium thioglycolate or ethanolamine thioglycolate	9–10	Quick processing time, tight curls	Harsh on hair shafts
Buffered alkaline	Ammonium bicarbonate added to alkaline curl ingredients	7–8.5	Less harsh on hair than alkaline perm	Less harsh than alkaline perm, but still damaging
Exothermic	Thioglycolate and peroxide to produce dithiodiglycolate	6.5–7	Heat produced for patient comfort	Must be properly mixed to prevent hair damage
Self-regulated	Dithioglycolic acid and thioglycolate	6.5–7	Stops processing automatically at equilibrium	Not good for hard-to-perm hair
Acid	Thioglycolate esters, such as glycerol monothioglycolate	6.5–7	Less damaging to hair	Produces looser, shorter-lasting curl
Sulfite	Sulfite or bisulfite	6–8	Less odor	Long processing time, harsh on hair

ammonium bicarbonate, is employed to reduce the pH to 7–8.5. This allows rapid production of a tight long-lasting curl with less hair damage.

Exothermic permanent waves

Another variation on the permanent wave, known as an exothermic permanent, is designed to increase patient comfort by reducing the chill from the cold waving solution. The heat is produced as a by-product of the chemical reaction when the oxidizing agent, such as hydrogen peroxide, is mixed with the thioglycolate-based waving lotion immediately prior to scalp application. The reaction of the thioglycolate with the peroxide produces dithiodiglycolate, the disulfide

of thioglycolate, which limits the extent to which the permanent wave can process. These products are only available for professional use, since irreversible hair damage can occur if the waving lotion is not properly mixed with the oxidizing agent prior to application.

Self-regulated permanent waves

One of the major problems for the hairstylist who performs permanent waves is getting to each client as soon as the processing time is completed. It is not unusual for a busy hairstylist to have three or four permanent waves processing at the same time. This need has led to the development of self-regulated permanent waves, designed to limit the amount of hair disulfide bond breakage. Overprocessing, due to leaving the permanent wave solution on the hair longer than recommended, causes extensive hair damage. If the permanent wave solution is left on the hair for an extended period of time, it can weaken the hair to the point that it may act like a depilatory, breaking all of the bonds such that the hair can be wiped away. Self-regulated permanent waves are designed to form a chemical equilibrium such that the disulfide bond breakage is stopped. This is accomplished by adding dithioglycolic acid to the thioglycolate-based waving lotion. This is the same chemical reaction discussed for exothermic permanent waves.

Acid permanent waves

Acid permanent waves, as opposed to alkaline permanent waves, are designed with an acidic waving lotion at a pH of 6.5–7. They are based on thioglycolate esters, such as glycerol monothioglycolate. The lower pH produces less hair shaft swelling, thus hair damage is minimized. These products result in a looser, shorter-lasting curl, but leave the hair soft. They are ideal for bleached or color-treated hair. It is possible to achieve a tighter curl if the permanent wave is processed with added heat under a hairdryer, but more hair shaft damage results. In general, tighter curls produce more hair damage and looser curls produce less hair damage.

Sulfite permanent waves

Sulfite permanent waves are mainly marketed for home use and have not found popularity among salons in the United States.

These products differ in that the reducing agent is a sulfite or bisulfite, instead of a mercaptan. This accounts for the reduced odor, which is their primary advantage. They require a long processing time at a pH of 6–8 and result in loose curls. A conditioning agent must be added to the formulation as the sulfite permanent waves can leave the hair feeling harsh.

Home permanents

Home permanents are designed for the non-professional and are of two types: ammonium thioglycolate permanents and sulfite permanents. The ammonium thioglycolate permanents have the same characteristics as the salon solutions except that they are one-third strength. This is to prevent excessive hair damage by the novice. Thus, home thioglycolate permanents produce looser curls that are not as long-lasting as salon permanents.

As mentioned previously, sulfite permanents are manufactured only for home use and have no professional counterpart. The major advantage of this type of permanent wave is decreased odor. The head is covered with a plastic cap to use body heat for processing and an alkaline rinse is applied as a neutralizer. The mild curls produced are not long-lasting.

DERMATOLOGIC CONSIDERATIONS

There are many changes that occur in the hair shaft following a permanent waving procedure.[13] These changes lead to some important dermatologic considerations. One of the key changes that occurs to the hair after permanent waving is a decrease in hair length. The dry waved hair shaft is shorter than the original hair shaft due to alterations in the disulfide bonds.[14] This may account for the perception by many patients that their hair was cut too short following a permanent waving procedure. Another important change is the loss of mechanical strength in the newly curled hair. The chemically treated hair shaft is 17% weaker and thus less able to withstand the trauma of combing and brushing.[15] This is due to actual hair protein loss from the permanent waving. Patients may comment that their hair is falling out following permanent waving when in actuality the hair shaft is fracturing more readily and breaking off. Thus, permanently waved hair shafts are both shortened and weakened.

Hair shortening and weakening is unavoidable, but there are several factors that determine the success or failure of a cold permanent waving procedure. Most of the suboptimal results that cause patients to seek dermatologic help result from failure to consider several key points while performing the procedure.[16] In this section, I shall present a common patient complaint, analyze the problem, and present a solution. The hope is that this discussion will help the dermatologist better address hair problems related to permanent waving procedures.

Concern #1
My hair keeps falling out after my permanent wave procedure.

In order to create the stress causing straight hair to reform into curls, the hair must be wound with tension around the curling rods. If the hair is wound with too much tension, excessive bond breaking occurs, weakening the hair shaft. Thus, the patient should be advised to suggest to her beautician that the hair not be wound as tightly around the curling rods.[17]

Concern #2
My hair does not curl tightly enough with a permanent wave and my beautician says I need a stronger perm.

The strength of the waving lotion does not determine the tightness of the curl. The degree of curl is determined by the diameter of the curling rods. Smaller rods produce smaller curls, but smaller curls are more damaging to the hair shaft. This patient should use the same strength waving solution, but smaller curling rods to avoid excessive hair shaft weakening.

Concern #3
I had a permanent wave, but my short hair did not curl.

In order to create a curl, the hair must fit around the curling rod one complete revolution. If the hair is too short, the curl will be incomplete. This patient should use smaller curling rods or let her hair grow longer. This is a common problem in mature women who get their hair cut short prior to undergoing a permanent waving procedure.

Concern #4
My permanent wave is tight for about one week and then loses the curl rapidly.

There is some loss of the new bond formation with water contact resulting in relaxation of the permanent wave. For this reason, most beauticians recommend that water contact and shampooing be avoided for at least 3 days following a permanent waving procedure. There is no doubt that the more the hair is washed, the more quickly the curl will be lost, especially in heavily damaged hair.

Concern #5
My hair gets dull and frizzy after a permanent waving procedure.

Hair that has been heavily damaged requires special care when undergoing a permanent waving procedure. The hair may have been heavily damaged from dyeing, bleaching, swimming, teasing, etc. In this case, the patient should ask her beautician to use a weak waving lotion combined with a shorter processing time. This will minimize excessive damage resulting in undue hair breakage.

Concern #6
My long hair is unattractive after a permanent waving procedure.

Hair that has been on the head for a longer period of time has experienced more cuticle scale loss simply because it has been manipulated for a longer period of time. This loss of cuticle scale allows the permanent waving solution to penetrate more thoroughly at the distal ends of the hair shaft than the proximal new growth. In this patient with long hair, it may be necessary to use different strengths of waving lotion. A stronger waving lotion can be used on the shorter cut hairs of the bangs and a weaker waving lotion on the longer more weathered hair.[18] This will optimize the degree of curl while minimizing hair damage.

Concern #7
My beautician wants to know how long she should leave the curling rods in my hair.

The typical way to determine how long the waving lotion should be left on the hair is to perform a test curl. Typically, the test curl is placed at the nape of the neck since this hair is more resistant to curling. However, in patients with damaged hair and hair breakage, it may be better to place the test curl at the anterior scalp. This hair typically has been manipulated more and has lost more cuticular scale. This test curl placement will prevent overprocessing of the anterior scalp

hair, but the curl may not be as tight at the posterior scalp. Sometimes a compromise of type is necessary to avoid excessive hair breakage.

Concern #8
My dyed hair changed color after my permanent wave procedure.

Hair should always undergo a permanent waving procedure first, followed by a dyeing procedure. Ideally, the two chemical procedures should be separated by at least 10 days. Hair discoloration may occur in patients who have used para-phenylenediamine-based permanent dyes that have been incompletely oxidized. Following these rules should avoid further problems.

Concern #9
My hair smells like rotten eggs ever since I had a permanent wave.

Patients who complain of an undesirable odor following permanent waving, especially after shampooing, have undergone incomplete neutralization. This means that some of disulfide bonds have not been rejoined and free sulfur is being released from the hair shafts. Repeating the neutralization process will reduce the excessive odor.[19] It is important to rejoin the disulfide bonds because failure to do so will result in excessive hair breakage from weakened hair shafts.

Concern #10
Permanent waves do not seem to work in my hair.

Some patients will note that a permanent wave does not 'take' in their hair. This means that the curl is short-lived. This may occur in patients who have rapidly growing hair. As the new proximal growth occurs, the curl is not as complete in the distal hair shaft and the appearance of the curled ringlets is lost. Patients with rapidly growing hair need to repeat the permanent waving procedure more frequently.

Concern #11
I am pregnant and my hair no longer seems to curl with a permanent wave.

Pregnancy is a time of extremely rapid hair growth. As discussed under concern #10, increased hair growth during pregnancy could account for the fact that some hairdressers note that permanent waves do not 'take' in pregnant women. Also, the new hair growth has a more intact cuticle and does not allow as thorough penetration of the waving lotion. A stronger waving lotion may need to be used during pregnancy. Permanent waves are felt to be safe for use in pregnant women.

Concern #12
The hair at the back of my head does not seem to curl.

Hair at the nape of the neck does not receive as much manipulation as hair around the face. For this reason, the cuticle is more intact in the hair at the posterior scalp than on the anterior scalp. This phenomenon is known as 'weathering' in the hair care industry. Weathered hair allows increased penetration of the waving lotion. Thus, the hair at the nape of the neck will not curl as readily due to the decreased penetration of the waving lotion. Taking the curling rods out of the anterior scalp first and out of the neck last can overcome this problem by allowing the waving solution to remain in contact with the rods at the nape of the neck for slightly longer.

Concern #13
My hair dries more slowly now that I have had it permanently waved.

Permanently waved hair does dry more slowly than natural hair. This is due to increased hair shaft swelling from cortical damage.[20] Unfortunately, this is an unavoidable side effect of the permanent waving procedure.

Concern #14
My hair dyes too darkly since my permanent wave procedure.

The increased hair shaft swelling and loss of the cuticle scale allow hair dyes to penetrate into the hair shaft more thoroughly. This can sometimes yield unpredictable results. It may be necessary to lighten the color of permanent hair dye selected to prevent undesirable hair darkening.

Concern #15
My hair is rough and hard to comb since I had it permanently waved.

Damage to the cuticle during the permanent waving process creates a roughened hair shaft surface. Thus, the hair demonstrates more frictional resistance following permanent waving.[21] This means it is more difficult to comb. Use of a silicone-based conditioner can help smooth the cuticular scale and increase ease of combing.

ADVERSE REACTIONS

The use of permanent wave solutions is considered safe; however, both irritant and allergic contact dermatitis to thioglycolate-containing waving lotions have been reported.[22] Irritant contact dermatitis is more common and can be avoided by minimizing skin contact with the permanent waving solution.[23] This is especially important in patients using topical tretinoin, who seem to experience skin irritation more readily with permanent waving. Prior to application of the waving lotion, a layer of petroleum jelly should be applied to the margins of the scalp and covered with a band of absorbent cotton. This provides a protective covering for the nonhair-bearing skin that might contact any waving lotion running over the scalp. Patients with sensitive scalp skin can even apply petroleum jelly to the scalp as protection. However, the petroleum jelly will limit the degree of curl achieved at the proximal hair shafts close to the scalp.

Allergic contact dermatitis can occur immediately after permanent waving or persist due to an allergen in the hair of patients who undergo permanent waving procedures involving glyceryl monothioglycolate (GMTG).[24,25] Glyceryl monothioglycolate is found in the acid permanent waving procedure previously discussed.[24] Interestingly enough, the hair may continue to be allergenic even after all products have been thoroughly rinsed from the hair. The North American Contact Dermatitis Group found this chemical to be the fifth most common cause of allergic contact dermatitis.[26] Glyceryl monothioglycolate can be patch tested at a 1% concentration in petrolatum, if allergy is suspected.[27]

REFERENCES

1. Lee AE, Bozza JB, Huff S, de la Mettrie R. Permanent waves: an overview. *Cosmet Toilet* 1988;**103**:37–56.
2. Wickett RR. Disulfide bond reduction in permanent waving. *Cosmet Toilet* 1991;**106**: 37–47.
3. Wickett RR. Permanent waving and straightening of hair. *Cutis* 1987;**39**:496–7.
4. Zviak C. Permanent waving and hair straightening. In: Zviak C, ed. *The science of hair care*. New York: Marcel Dekker, 1986:183–209.
5. Cannell DW. Permanent waving and hair straightening. *Clin Dermatol* 1988;**6**:71–82.
6. Busch P, Thiele D, Fischer D, Hollenberg D. Testing permanent waves. *Cosmet Toilet* 1996;**111**:41–54.
7. Heilingotter R. Permanent waving of hair. In: de Navarre MG, ed. *The chemistry and manufacture of cosmetics*. Wheaton, IL: Allured Publishing, 1988:1167–227.
8. Shipp JJ. Hair-care products. In: *Chemistry and technology of the cosmetics and toiletries industry*. London: Blackie Academic & Professional, 1992:80–6.
9. Szadurski JS, Erlemann G. The hair loop test – a new method of evaluating perm lotions. *Cosmet Toilet* 1984;**99**:41–6.
10. Draelos ZK. Hair cosmetics. *Dermatol Clin* 1991;**9**:19–27.
11. Ishihara M. The composition of hair preparations and their skin hazards. In: Koboir T, Montagna W, eds. *Biology and disease of the hair*. Baltimore: University Park Press, 1975:603–29.
12. Gershon SD, Goldberg MA, Rieger MM. Permanent waving. In: Balsam MS, Sagarin E, eds. *Cosmetics science and technology*, Vol 2, 2nd edn. New York: Wiley-Interscience, John Wiley & Sons, 1972:167–250.
13. Kon R, Nakamura A, Hirabayashi N, Takeuchi K. Analysis of the damaged components of permed hair using biochemical technique. *J Cosmet Sci* 1998;**49**:13–22.
14. Garcia ML, Nadgorny EM, Wolfram LJ. Letter to the Editor. *J Soc Cosmet Chem* 1990;**41**:149–54.
15. Feughelman M. A note on the permanent setting of human hair. *J Soc Cosmet Chem* 1990;**41**:209–12.
16. Heilingotter R. Permanent waving of hair. In: de Navarre MG ed. *The chemistry and manufacture of cosmetics*. Wheaton, IL: Allured Publishing, 1988:1167–227.
17. Wortman FJ, Souren I. Extensional properties of human hair and permanent waving. *J Soc Cosmet Chem* 1987;**38**:125–40.
18. Inoue T, Ito M, Kizawa K. Labile proteins accumulated in damaged hair upon permanent waving and bleaching treatments. *J Cosmet Sci* 2002;**53**:337–44.

19. Brunner MJ. Medical aspects of home cold waving. *Arch Dermatol* 1952;**65**:316–26.

20. Shansky A. The osmotic behavior of hair during the permanent waving process as explained by swelling measurements. *J Soc Cosmet Chem* 1963;**14**:427–32.

21. Robbins CR. *Chemical and physical behavior of human hair*. New York: Springler-Verlag, 1988:94–8.

22. Lehman AJ. Health aspects of common chemicals used in hair-waving preparations. *JAMA* 1949;**141**:842–5.

23. Fisher AA. Management of hairdressers sensitized to hair dyes or permanent wave solutions. *Cutis* 1989;**43**:316–18.

24. Morrison LH, Storrs FJ. Persistence of an allergen in hair after glyceryl monothioglycolate-containing permanent wave solutions. *J Am Acad Dermatol* 1988;**19**:52–9.

25. Storrs FJ. Permanent wave contact dermatitis: contact allergy to glyceryl monothioglycolate. *J Am Acad Dermatol* 1984;**11**:74–85.

26. Adams RM, Maibach HI. A five-year study of cosmetic reactions. *J Am Acad Dermatol* 1985;**13**:1062–9.

27. White IR, Rycroft RJG, Anderson KE *et al*. The patch test dilution of glyceryl thioglycolate. *Contact Dermatitis* 1990;**23**:198–9.

6 Permanent hair straightening

Hair straightening is a common practice among individuals with kinky hair.[1] The hair can be straightened with heat or chemical techniques.[2] Heat straightening techniques are temporary and have already been covered on page 67. This chapter discusses the permanent method of hair straightening, also known as lanthionization. Hair straightening is undertaken for many reasons including those listed in Box 6.1.[3]

The first permanent hair straighteners, also known as hair relaxers or perms, were developed around 1940 and consisted of sodium hydroxide or potassium hydroxide mixed into potato starch. Once the disulfide bonds were broken, the hair was pulled straight and the disulfide bonds reformed in their new configuration. This chapter examines the physical and chemical differences between African-American hair and Caucasian hair, discusses the chemistry of hair straightening, reviews the unique aspects of the hair straightening techniques, and presents the relevant dermatologic considerations.

CHARACTERISTICS

There are some unique differences between Caucasian hair and African-American hair. These differences have already been discussed on page 7. Table 6.1 summarizes some of the key differences.[4] It is interesting

---

Box 6.1 Rationale for permanent hair straightening

1. Hair manageability is improved
2. The hair can be more easily combed and styled
3. Hair breakage may be decreased due to less combing friction
4. Hair shine is improved with a straighter hair shaft
5. Fashion may dictate the need for straight hair
6. Versatility in straightening techniques allows multiple styling options: completely straightened, minimally straightened, texturized, or straightened and recurled

Table 6.1 Comparative physical characteristics of African-American hair

Property evaluated	African-American	Caucasian	Asian
Maximum length (mm)	15–30	60–100	100–150
Thickness	High	Medium	Low
Shape	Kidney	Oval	Round
Force (g)	33	43	63
Breaking strength dry (N/m^2)	0.153	0.189	
Breaking strength wet (N/m^2)	0.089	0.165	
Elongation at breaking point – wet (%)	42	62	
Elongation at breaking point – dry (%)	39	50	

Adapted from Vermeulen S, Banham A, Brooks G. Ethnic hair care. *Cosmet Toilet* 2002;**117**:69–78.

to note that African-American hair has a greater thickness but requires less strength to break than Caucasian hair. Notice that Asian hair grows the longest and is the most resistant to breakage. This may account for the fact that most human hair wigs for African-Americans are woven from treated Asian hair. There are also subtle amino acid, sulfur, and ammonia differences between African-American and Caucasian hair (Table 6.2).

In summary, it can be said that African-American hair has fewer cuticle layers than Caucasian hair, 7 as compared to 12. The hair shafts have a larger diameter, but tend to break where the hair begins to kink at pinch points.[5] Lastly, African-American hair has a lower moisture content than Caucasian hair, reducing hair shaft elasticity and encouraging breakage.

CHEMISTRY

Hair relaxing, also known as lanthionization, is a chemical process whereby extremely curly hair is straightened through the use of metal hydroxides, such as sodium, lithium, potassium, or guanidine hydroxide, to change about 35% of the cysteine contents of the hair to lanthionine along with minor hydrolysis of the peptide bonds.[6] Chemical relaxing can be accomplished with lye-based, lye-free, ammonium thioglycolate, or bisulfite creams.[7]

Lye-based, or sodium hydroxide straighteners are alkaline creams with a pH of 13. Sodium hydroxide is a caustic substance that can damage hair, produce scalp burns, and cause blindness if exposed to the eye. These products are generally restricted to professional or salon use and may contain up to 3.5% sodium hydroxide. The basic chemistry of hair relaxing with lye products is depicted in Box 6.2 while the hair rearrangement schematic is presented in Figure 6.1.[8]

Lye relaxers are available in 'base' and 'no-base' forms (Box 6.3). The 'base' is usually petrolatum that is applied to the scalp and hairline prior to application of the sodium hydroxide. This prevents scalp irritation and burns. The 'base' relaxers contain between 1.5% and 3.5% sodium hydroxide

Table 6.2 Comparative chemical amino acid characteristics of African-American and Caucasian hair

Amino acids and other hair components	African-American hair content	Caucasian hair content
Glycine	541	539
Alanine	509	471
Valine	568	538
Leucine	570	554
Isoleucine	277	250
Serine	672	870
Threonine	615	653
Tyrosine	202	132
Phenylalanine	179	130
Aspartic acid	436	455
Glutamic acid	915	871
Lysine	23	213
Arginine	482	512
Histidine	84	63
Sulfur	1380	1440
Half cystine	1370	1380
Cysteic acid	10	55
Proline	662	672
Ammonia	935	780

Adapted from Vermeulen S, Banham A, Brooks G. Ethnic hair care. *Cosmet Toilet* 2002;**117**:69–78.

Box 6.2 Chemistry of hair relaxing

Strong alkali chemical relaxing

$NaOH + K\text{-}S\text{-}S\text{-}K\ \underline{OH\text{-}}\ K\text{-}S\text{-}K + Na_2S + H_2O$

(alkali can be Na+, K+, or Li+)

Chemical reaction that occurs with a guanidine hydroxide product.

Adapted from Obukowho P, Birman M. Hair curl relaxers: a discussion of their function, chemistry, and manufacture. *Cosmet Toilet* 1995;**110**:65–9.

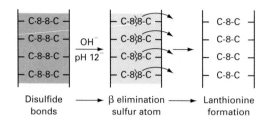

Figure 6.1
Schematic of hair straightening bond rearrangement. (Adapted from Obukowho P, Birman M. Hair curl relaxers: a discussion of their function, chemistry, and manufacture. *Cosmet Toilet* 1995;**110**:65–9.)

Box 6.4 Ingredients in a no-lye cream relaxer

Cream relaxer components
Petrolatum
Mineral oil
Fatty alcohol
Emulsifying wax
Simethicone
Water
Propylene glycol
Calcium hydroxide

Liquid activator components
Water
Propylene glycol
Xanthan gum
Guanidine carbonate

and therefore require that the scalp and hairline be coated with a petrolatum base prior to application. These higher concentration lye products are necessary for hard-to-straighten hair. 'No-base' relaxers, on the other hand, contain 1.5%–2.5% sodium hydroxide and only require base application to the hairline.[9] They are more popular, because it is time-consuming for the beautician to apply the base to the scalp and most individuals are re-straightening hair that has already been chemically weakened.

Other strong alkali chemicals sometimes used in place of sodium hydroxide are

guanidine hydroxide and lithium hydroxide, which are known as 'no-lye' chemical hair straighteners (Box 6.4). These relaxing kits contain 4–7% cream calcium hydroxide and liquid guanidine carbonate. The guanidine carbonate activator is then mixed into the calcium hydroxide cream to produce calcium carbonate and guanidine hydroxide, the active agent. These products do not require basing of either the scalp or the hairline. The chemical reaction that occurs with a guanidine hydroxide product is illustrated in Figure 6.2.

Table 6.3 compares the lye and no-lye relaxers in terms of their effect on the hair shaft.

Thioglycolate can also be used as an active agent in hair straightening.[10] These are the same thioglycolate chemicals that were described as permanent wave solutions in Chapter 5, except that they are formulated as thick creams, rather than lotions. The cream adds weight to hair and helps to pull it straight. Also, instead of the hair being wound on mandrels, it is combed straight

Box 6.3 Ingredients in a lye no-base relaxer

Petrolatum
Mineral oil
Fatty alcohol
Emulsifying wax
Simethicone
Water
Propylene glycol
Sodium lauryl sulfate
Sodium hydroxide (lye)

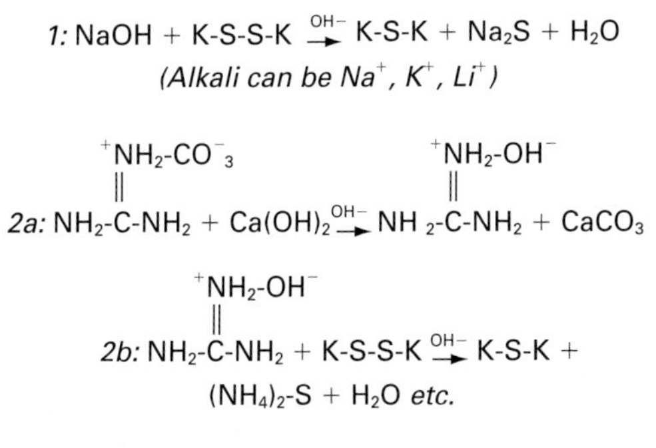

1: $NaOH + K\text{-}S\text{-}S\text{-}K \xrightarrow{OH^-} K\text{-}S\text{-}K + Na_2S + H_2O$

(Alkali can be Na^+, K^+, Li^+)

2a: $NH_2\text{-}\overset{\overset{+NH_2\text{-}CO^-_3}{\|}}{C}\text{-}NH_2 + Ca(OH)_2 \xrightarrow{OH^-} NH_2\text{-}\overset{\overset{+NH_2\text{-}OH^-}{\|}}{C}\text{-}NH_2 + CaCO_3$

2b: $NH_2\text{-}\overset{\overset{+NH_2\text{-}OH^-}{\|}}{C}\text{-}NH_2 + K\text{-}S\text{-}S\text{-}K \xrightarrow{OH^-} K\text{-}S\text{-}K +$

$(NH_4)_2\text{-}S + H_2O$ etc.

Figure 6.2
Chemical reaction that occurs with a guanidine hydroxide product. (Adapted from Obukowho P, Birman M. Hair curl relaxers: a discussion of their function, chemistry, and manufacture. *Cosmet Toilet* 1995;**110**:65–9.)

while the thioglycolate cream is in contact with the hair shaft. Thioglycolate hair straighteners are extremely harsh on the hair and are the least popular of all the relaxing chemicals for this reason. The thioglyco-late cream has a pH of 9.0–9.5, which removes the protective sebum and facilitates hair shaft penetration. Chemical burns can also occur with this variety of chemical hair straightener.[11]

The least damaging of all hair straightening chemicals are the ammonium bisulfite creams. These products contain a mixture of bisulfite and sulfite in varying ratios depending on the pH of the lotion. Many of the home chemical straightening products are of this type, but can only produce short-lived straightening. These are very similar to the home sulfite permanent waves discussed in Chapter 5, except here again the hair is combed straight instead of being wound on curling rods.

As a general rule, the chemicals that produce the greatest, longest-lasting hair straightening are also the most damaging to the hair shaft. Box 6.5 presents the important considerations when selecting a relaxer product.

Table 6.3 Comparison of lye and no-lye chemical relaxers

Hair quality	Lye chemical relaxer	No-lye chemical relaxer
Relative strength on scale of 1–3 (higher number is stronger)	3	1
Alkaline relaxing agent	NaOH or KOH	Guanidine hydroxide
Chemical agent	OH	OH
pH	12.5–14	12.5–13.5
Hair shaft penetration	Faster	Slower
Processing time	Shorter	Longer
Irritation	High	Low
Hair-drying potential	Less drying to hair and scalp	More drying to hair and scalp

Adapted from Obukowho P, Birman M. Hair curl relaxers: a discussion of their function, chemistry, and manufacture. *Cosmet Toilet* 1995;**110**:65–9.

Box 6.5 Considerations for selecting a hair relaxer

1. Relaxer must effectively straighten hair
2. Relaxer must contain adequate petrolatum and other oils to protect against scalp and hairline irritation
3. Relaxer must be stable at room temperature
4. Relaxer must be an easy to apply cream that spreads over hair with sufficient weight to pull hair straight
5. Relaxer must rinse easily with warm water
6. Relaxer must not damage hair beyond acceptable limits

APPLICATION TECHNIQUE FOR HAIR RELAXING

This chapter has presented the basic chemistry involved in hair relaxing and now presents the application technique. Whether the patient chooses to utilize lye-based, no-lye, thioglycolate, or sulfite chemicals to induce the straightening, the application technique is similar (Box 6.6).[12] Shampooing is the first step in the permanent waving technique for straight hair, but the hair is not shampooed when straightening is undertaken. This is because hair straightening chemicals are far more irritating and shampooing would remove the protective sebum from the scalp. As a matter of fact, the protective sebum is supplemented with a petrolatum base applied to the scalp and hairline to prevent skin burns (Figure 6.3). Following application of the base, the hair is divided into quadrants allowing the hair stylist to work systematically (Figure 6.4). For previously untreated hair, the chemical straightener is applied from hair root to distal end beginning at the nape of the neck and moving forward to the anterior hairline (Figures 6.5 and 6.6). The hair at the nape of the neck receives the chemical first, since it is subject to less weathering, resulting in the presence

---

Box 6.6 Hair relaxing steps

1. Do not shampoo
2. Apply petrolatum base to scalp and hairline
3. Section hair
4. Apply cream relaxer from hair root to end beginning at nape of neck
5. Gently comb hair straight for 10–30 minutes until degree of relaxation is achieved
6. Rinse thoroughly with water
7. Apply neutralizer
8. Shampoo
9. Apply conditioner
10. Style
11. Apply styling conditioner

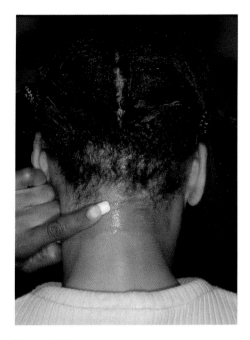

Figure 6.3
A petrolatum base is applied to the entire hairline and scalp.

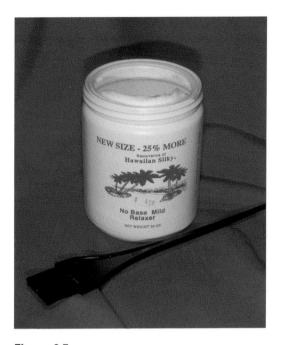

Figure 6.5
The cream straightening product is packaged in a jar.

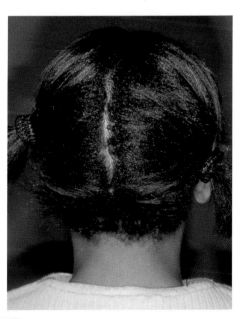

Figure 6.4
The hair is divided by parting into quadrants.

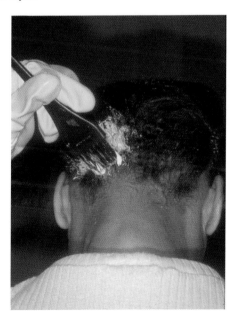

Figure 6.6
The cream is scooped from the jar and applied to the scalp with a stiff brush.

of more cuticular scale (Figure 6.7). This means it will be more resistant to the lanthionization process. The chemicals are left in contact with the hair for only 20–30 minutes, during which time the hairstylist is combing the hair straight (Figure 6.8). The hairstylist must wear gloves and work quickly to get the straightening cream worked through all areas of the scalp (Figure 6.9). Longer contact of the chemicals with the hair shafts will result in irreversible damage.

For previously treated hair, the chemical straightener is applied to the new growth only, taking care to minimize scalp contact. Usually the straightening cream is applied to the hair closest to the scalp first and then combed through the previously relaxed distal ends for the last 10 minutes of the process (Figure 6.10). The hair is combed to pull it straight concurrently with the straightening cream application (Figure 6.11). The

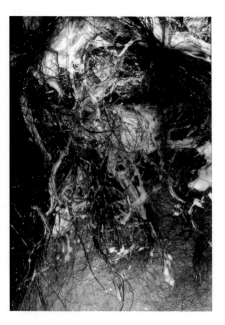

Figure 6.8
The straightener is applied to the hair next to the scalp over the entire head.

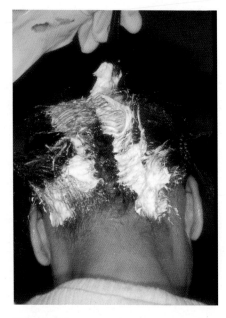

Figure 6.7
Application of the straightener to the hair close to the scalp at the nape of the neck.

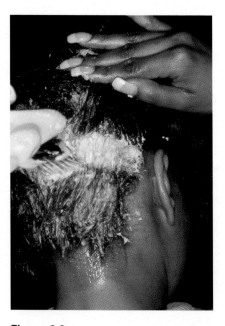

Figure 6.9
A protective rubber glove is worn to prevent the strong alkali from producing cutaneous burns.

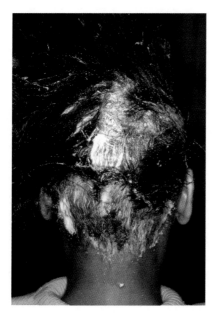

Figure 6.10
The relaxer has been applied to
the entire scalp within 10 minutes.

hairstylist should completely remove all of the straightening chemicals within 20 minutes. This requires skill and organization. It is for this reason that hair straightening should not be attempted by someone without education and experience.

When the hair has relaxed to the desired degree of straightening, the cream must be thoroughly removed by rinsing with water. A neutralizer is then smoothed on the hair, taking care to keep it straight and untangled, since the hair shafts can very easily fracture until the neutralization process is complete (Figure 6.12). Once the hair has been thoroughly neutralized, it is shampooed with a nonalkaline shampoo to minimize hair shaft swelling (Figure 6.13). A conditioner must be applied immediately following shampooing to decrease water loss from the hair shaft (Figure 6.14). The hair straightening chemicals produce holes in the hair shaft cuticle through which the

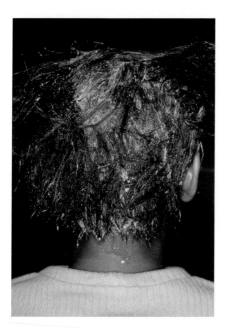

Figure 6.11
The hair is combed and pulled
straight.

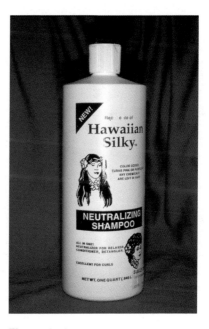

Figure 6.12
The neutralizer lotion.

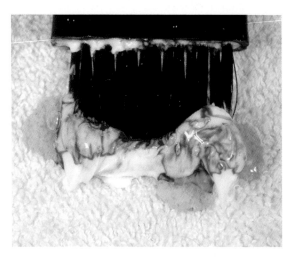

Figure 6.13
The neutralizer has a pH indicator and turns pink when applied to any hair that still contains the alkaline lye.

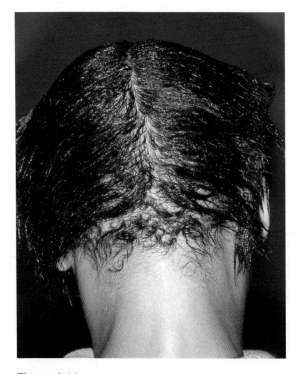

Figure 6.14
The hair has been shampooed and conditioned.

hair shaft water evaporates, leaving the hair shaft dry and inelastic. The remoisturizing post-straightening conditioner minimizes hair shaft brittleness and breakage. The formulation presented in Box 6.7 contains panthenol as a humectant, dicetyldimonium chloride as a conditioner, cetearyl alcohol and mineral oil as emollients, and octyl dimethyl PABA as a UV protectant. The hair is then dried and styled (Figure 6.15). Following styling, a second conditioner is applied to further condition the hair shafts. The formulation presented in Box 6.8 contains petrolatum, mineral oil, and beeswax to prevent water loss and add hair shaft shine.

There are two other styling variations of hair relaxers known as blow-out relaxers and texturizing relaxers. The chemicals employed and the lanthionization process are identical to those previously discussed. The blow-out relaxers minimally straighten the hair shaft leaving it more manageable, but preserving some of the curl. Texturizing relaxers leave the hair wavy and not completely straight (Figure 6.16). Both of these relaxer varieties are most popular among men with short hair.

Box 6.7 Remoisturizing post-straightening conditioner

Water
Methylpraben
Imidazolidinyl urea
Panthenol
Sodium PCA
Cetearyl alcohol
Dicetyldimonium chloride
Mineral oil
Polysorbate-20
Propylparaben
Octyl dimethyl PABA
Fragrance

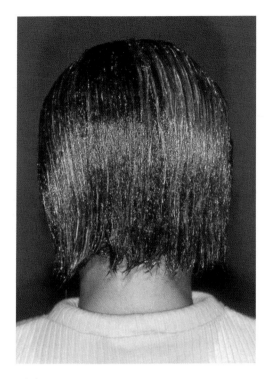

Figure 6.15
The appearance of the newly straightened hair.

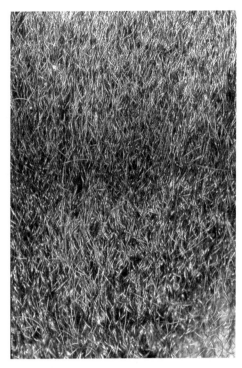

Figure 6.16
The appearance of texturized hair.

Box 6.8 Oil moisturizing lotion styling conditioner

Petrolatum
Mineral oil
Propylparaben
Beeswax
Stearic hydrazide
Sorbitan sesquioleate
Polysorbate-80
Water
Methylparaben
Imidazolidinyl urea
Sodium borate
Fragrance

The key to successful hair relaxing is an experienced beautician who can quickly apply and remove the chemicals and determine when the desired degree of disulfide bond breaking has occurred. It is estimated that virgin hair loses about 30% of its tensile strength following a properly performed chemical straightening procedure. It also becomes more porous, allowing future relaxing procedures to process more quickly.[13] Hair relaxing is a careful balance between achieving the straightening of kinky hair and minimizing irreversible hair shaft damage (Figure 6.17).

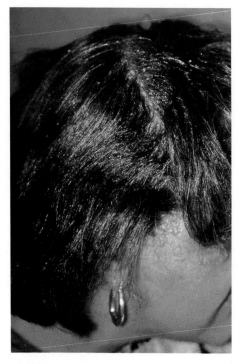

Figure 6.17
The appearance of relaxed hair.

APPLICATION TECHNIQUE FOR HAIR PERMING

Another technique for relaxing kinky hair is known as hair perming. The products used are similar to Caucasian permanent waves, in that they are based on ammonium thioglycolate, which is neutralized with ammonium hydroxide. The main differences between a straight hair perm and a kinky hair perm are the level of the active ingredients and the application technique. Perming is performed in four stages consisting of rearranging, boosting, neutralizing, and conditioning (Box 6.9).

Permanent waving of kinky hair begins by shampooing and sectioning the hair as described for hair straightening. A cream is then applied containing high levels of ammonium thioglycolate in the range of 7–7.5%. This cream is known as the reducing cream or rearranger. It is applied from the hair root to distal end on virgin hair starting at the nape of the neck proceeding to the anterior hair line. In previously chemically treated hair, the rearranger is only applied to new growth. Its purpose is to straighten the hair in preparation for the curling procedure. The rearranger is then rinsed and a reducing lotion or curl booster is applied from the hair root to the distal end. The hair is then sectioned and wrapped around perming rods. The patient is placed under a hooded hairdryer to increase the rate of the chemical reaction with heat. After 15–20 minutes, a test curl is performed to determine if the desired amount of curl has been obtained. This is assessed by unwrapping several rods and observing if the hair makes a complete 'S', meaning that the desired amount of curl has been achieved. This is identical to the reducing step in a permanent wave on straight hair. The hair is then thoroughly rinsed.

Next the hair is ready for neutralization with an oxidizing solution containing 10–13% sodium bromate for 15–20 minutes. This sets the curls and the rods are removed. The hair is then thoroughly rinsed. A variety of conditioners and glycerin curl activators are now applied to prevent excessive hair shaft water loss and hair brittleness. The hair is then dried and styled as desired.

These kinky hair perm products, known as the 'Jheri' curl after the company that pioneered the technology, were introduced in the late 1970s. They have recently lost some of their original appeal as the curling procedure is extremely damaging to African-American hair, leaving it frizzy, dry, and brittle. Daily use of propylene glycol and glycerin curl activators is required prior to styling to maintain the hairstyle and decrease breakage. Unfortunately, the glyc-

---

Box 6.9 Kinky hair permanent waving technique

1. Shampoo hair
2. Section hair into quadrants
3. Apply rearranger from hair root to distal hair shaft starting with hair at the nape of the neck and moving forward
4. Rinse rearranger with water
5. Apply booster from hair root to distal hair shaft starting with the hair at the nape of the neck and moving forward
6. Section hair
7. Wrap hair around rods
8. Place patient under hooded hairdryer for 15–20 minutes
9. Perform test curl
10. Rinse hair thoroughly
11. Apply neutralizer to each rod for 15–20 minutes
12. Remove curling rods
13. Rinse hair thoroughly
14. Apply conditioner for 10–20 minutes
15. Dry hair
16. Apply glycerin curl activator
17. Style hair

---

erin styling products leave the hair sticky and tend to stain clothing and pillowcases. It is also necessary to repeat the procedure every 12 weeks, further weakening the hair shafts and predisposing to hair loss through breakage.

Unless a severe chemical burn has occurred, which is unusual, hair straightening does not damage the follicle (Figure 6.18). Hair breakage is most commonly the cause of hair loss. The dermatologist can verify hair breakage by noting that the lost hairs do not

DERMATOLOGIC CONSIDERATIONS

Kinky hair that has been overprocessed by use of strong chemical straightener or an excessively long processing time will lose its elastic properties. The hair shafts become brittle, fracturing with minimal combing trauma usually at the scalp, where stress is maximal. Patients frequently comment that their hair is falling out following an aggressive chemical straightening procedure.

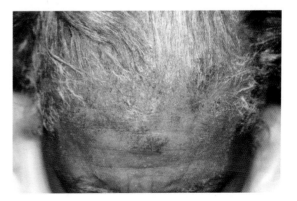

Figure 6.18
A chemical burn due to hair relaxing.

include the hair bulb. Unfortunately, if the hair has been appropriately neutralized, there is nothing that can be done to repair the damaged disulfide bonds. The brittle hair must be trimmed and overprocessing of the new growth should be avoided. Hair breakage can be minimized by combing or styling the hair as little as possible, applying moisturizing conditioning agents, and avoiding any further chemical treatments such as permanent hair dyeing or bleaching.[14]

ADVERSE REACTIONS

Hair straightening chemicals are all well-known cutaneous irritants. It is for this reason that a petrolatum cream is applied as a base to the scalp and hairline. They are not suitable for patch testing. Chemical burns are possible if a novice is performing the straightening procedure. This is why hair straightening should be performed in a salon by a trained professional to avoid adverse reactions.

REFERENCES

1. Bernard B. Hair shape of curly hair. *J Am Acad Dermatol* 2003;48(Suppl):S120–S126.
2. McDonald CJ. Special requirements in cosmetics for people with black skin. In: Frost P, Horwitz SN, eds. *Principles of cosmetics for the dermatologist*. St Louis: CV Mosby, 1982:302–4.
3. Syed A, Kuhajda A, Ayoub H, Ahmad K. African-American Hair. *Cosmet Toilet* 1995;**110**:39–48.
4. Franbourg A, Hallegot P, Baltenneck F, Toutain C, Leroy F. Current research on ethnic hair. J Am Acad Dermatol 2003;**48**(Suppl): S115-S119.
5. McMichael A. Ethnic hair update: past and present. *J Am Acad Dermatol* 2003;**48**: S127–S133.
6. Hsuing DY. Hair straightening. In: de Navarre MG, ed. *The chemistry and manufacture of cosmetics*, 2nd ed. Wheaton, IL: Allured Publishing, 1975: 1155–66
7. Cannell DW. Permanent waving and hair straightening. *Clin Dermatol* 1988;**6**:71–82.
8. Syed A. Ethnic hair care: history, trends, and formulation. *Cosmet Toilet* 1993;**108**: 99–108.
9. Khalil EN. Cosmetic and hair treatments for the black consumer. *Cosmet Toilet* 1986;**101**: 51–8.
10. Ogawa S, Fufii K, Kaneyama K, Arai K, Joko K. A curing method for permanent hair straightening using thioglycolic and dithiodiglycolic acids. *J Cosmet Sci* 2000;**51**: 379–99.
11. Bulengo R, Bergfeld WF. Chemical and traumatic alopecia from thioglycolate in a black woman. Cutis 1992;**49**:99–103.
12. Brooks G. Treatment regimes for styled black hair. Cosmet Toilet 1983;**98**:59–68.
13. Syed A, Ayoub H. Correlating porosity and tensile strength of chemically modified hair. *Cosmet Toilet* 2002;**117**:57–62.
14. Burmeister F, Bollatti D, Brooks G. Ethnic hair: moisturizing after relaxer use. Cosmet Toilet 1991;**106**:49–51.

7 Cosmetic-induced hair loss

Dermatologists are frequently confronted by both male and female patients who are concerned about hair loss. This hair loss may be due to medical concerns, a topic discussed in Chapter one of this text, or to the improper use of hair cosmetics. This chapter outlines a methodology for assessing the condition of the hair to determine if the hair loss is due to excessive hair breakage, in actuality the most common cause of hair loss. It then undertakes a discussion of the causes of cosmetic-induced hair loss followed by treatment suggestions. Even in the patient experiencing medically related hair loss, hair breakage is still an issue. Preventing hair breakage is of great cosmetic importance since the hair is a nonliving, slowly renewable protein fiber.

METHOD FOR ASSESSING HAIR CONDITION

Assessing the patient's scalp for cosmetic hair damage is best done with the naked eye and the fingers. The eye can observe the shine, color, degree of curl, length, and overall appearance of the hair while the fingers can assess hair softness. The assessment is best performed in an orderly fashion, asking the appropriate questions to collect information that will lead to a final diagnosis and ultimately a treatment recommendation. The questions that should be asked for a cosmetic hair assessment are listed in Box 7.1. Each of these assessments is discussed in detail.

Does the hair have shine?

Hair shine is visually assessed by looking at the amount of light reflection from the hair.[1] Healthy hair has high shine representing an intact cuticle with closely overlapping cuticular scales. It is the smoothness of the overlapping scales that promotes light reflection, interpreted by the eye as shine.[2] Normal grooming processes such as combing and brushing result in loss of cuticular scales, which is more pronounced at the distal hair shaft.[3] This process is known as 'weathering' and is accelerated by overly aggressive grooming and chemical processing[4,5] (Figure 7.1). Hair shine is also decreased in kinky hair found in African-American patients due to the naturally irregular nature of the shape of the hair shaft.[6]

Box 7.1 Cosmetic hair assessment methodology

1. Does the hair have shine?
2. Does the hair feel soft?
3. Does the hair lay in an orderly fashion?
4. Is there evidence of hairstyling aid use?
5. Does the hair color appear natural and match the patient's eyebrows, eyelashes, and body hair?
6. Is the hair curly or straight?
7. How long is the hair and when was it last cut?
8. Is there evidence of heat damage to the hair shaft?

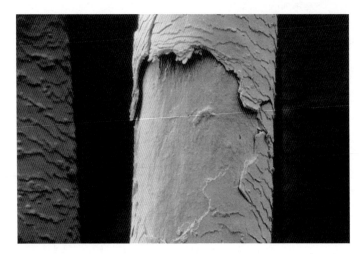

Figure 7.1
An electron micrograph of weathering manifested by cuticle loss.

Hair that is characterized by decreased or absent cuticular scales is dull, harsh, and frizzy. If the cuticular scales are greatly decreased at the distal hair shaft, the weak medulla is exposed and the hair splits, a condition known medically as trichoptilosis. Split ends result in frizzy, unmanageable hair (Figure 7.2). Sometimes cuticular loss can be combined with hair twisting and knotting, a condition known medically as trichonodosis.

Does the hair feel soft?

Hair shine is a visual assessment of the state of the cuticle while hair softness is a tactile assessment of the cuticle. An intact cuticle creates a smooth hair shaft surface which can be appreciated as hair softness. Permanently waved or dyed hair must have a disrupted cuticle in order to allow penetration of the waving lotion or dye. Thus, chemically processed hair never feels as soft as virgin hair, even though hair conditioners attempt to temporarily smooth the disrupted

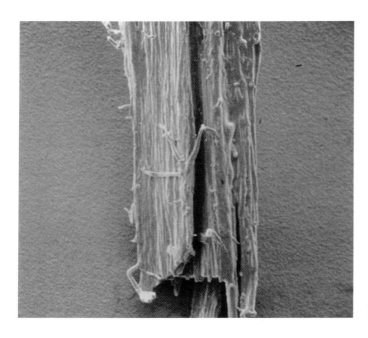

Figure 7.2
An electron micrograph
demonstrating trichoptilosis.

cuticle. Hair that feels harsh is evidence of severe cuticular damage (Figure 7.3).

Does the hair lay in an orderly fashion?

Hair that has a disrupted cuticle not only appears dull and feels harsh, but is also subject to the effects of static electricity. This is most apparent in hair that has been chemically processed either through dyeing or permanent waving procedures. Static electricity allows the hair to appear frizzy and unruly, especially at the distal hair shafts. This is because the hair shafts repel each other due to similar electrical charges. Generally, chemicals applied to the hair penetrate better at the distal hair shaft due to less cuticular scale. A well educated cosmetologist is aware of this fact, especially when processing long hair, and will apply the chemicals to the scalp first and then dilute the product prior to applying the solutions to the distal hair shafts. Overprocessed hair appears frizzy and is severely weakened and can never be restored to its original configuration. Static electricity is one manifestation of irreversible hair shaft damage.

Is there evidence of hairstyling aid use?

Styling aids can cover up some of the cuticle damage previously discussed. They can restore shine, add softness, and decrease static electricity. It is important for the physician not to be misled when evaluating hair covered with styling aids such as hairspray, mousse, or sculpturing gel. These products contain polymers which form a thin film over the hair shafts, imparting an improved cosmetic appearance. Combing the hair will remove the polymer film, which will appear as tiny white flakes throughout the hair, but the true state of the hair shafts can be better appreciated.

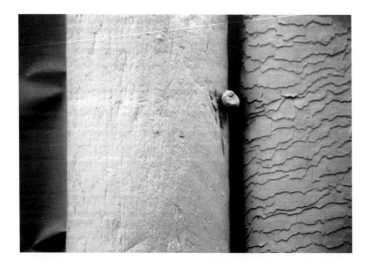

Figure 7.3
The electron micrographic
appearance of hair that feels harsh.

Does the hair color appear natural and match the patient's eyebrows, eyelashes, and body hair?

Unfortunately, some patients who dye their hair will not openly admit that they use hair coloring. Furthermore, many patients do not know what kind of dye has been applied to the hair and whether any bleaching has occurred. This means that the physician makes an assessment based on guided observation. The hair color should be compared to eyelashes, eyebrows, or other body hair. If the scalp hair color is lighter than other hair, bleaching has occurred. If regrowth is present at the scalp, a permanent hair color has been used. If the color appears to vary gradually from the proximal hair shaft to the distal hair shaft with the presence of some grayish hairs, a semipermanent hair color has been used. If the hair has a yellowish cast, a metallic hair color has been used. These guidelines can be used to initiate conversation when obtaining a patient history.

It is also important to note how different the patient's scalp hair color is from the rest of the body hair. The greater the difference in color, the more damage the hair shafts have sustained. The most damaging form of hair coloring is bleaching the hair to a lighter shade. Bleaching severely weakens the hair shafts making them more susceptible to hair breakage. With repeated bleaching, especially bleaching of selected hairs, patients will say that their hair is no longer 'taking' the bleached hair color. In actuality, the hairs are bleaching successfully, they are just selectively breaking off such that only the unbleached hairs and the unbleached hair color is left. Patients who bleach their hair extensively may also comment that their hair is not growing. This too is related to hair breakage that exceeds hair growth overall resulting in shortening of the hair shafts. It is important for the physician to assess hair loss in the context of chemical processing.

Is the hair curly or straight?

In addition to the color, the curl of the hair should also be assessed, since tightly curled hair is more prone to breakage. It should also be determined whether the curl is natural or due to permanent waving. Hair that has been chemically waved appears straight at the scalp and curlier at the ends. Hair that is naturally curly will have an even curl throughout the length of the hair shaft. If the hair has been chemically waved, the type of permanent wave and length of processing should be obtained either from the patient or from the salon. These factors cannot be determined by visual examination.

There are several common problems associated with permanent waving of the hair besides hair breakage. One is an irregular, uneven curl. This is typically due to failure to wrap the hair evenly on the mandrels with consistent tension. Figure 7.4 demonstrates the proper even wrapping technique and careful placement of the curling mandrels over the scalp. It is also important not to have loose hair ends sticking out of the mandrels (Figure 7.5). Any hairs that are not wound around the mandrel will remain straight, leading to an uneven appearance of the hair. This unevenness will contribute to decreased shine and lack of hair softness.

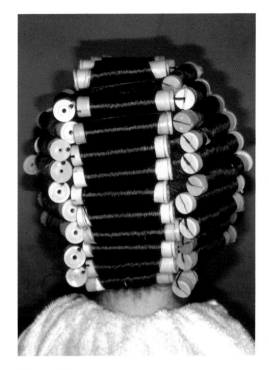

Figure 7.4
Proper placement of permanent waving mandrels.

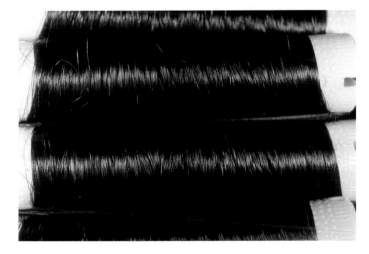

Figure 7.5
Proper technique for wrapping hair over the curling mandrel.

How long is the hair and when was it last cut?

The length of the hair is also important. Longer hair naturally will have been present on the scalp longer and would be expected to be more weathered and subject to increased breakage. The distal ends of the longer hair shafts may also be lighter in color and weaker due to photodegradation.[7] Patients frequently evaluate the number of hairs they are losing by the amount present in the sink. Longer hair shafts will create a larger lump than shorter hair shafts even though the same number of hairs have been lost. Thus, patients with longer hair tend to overestimate their actual loss.

The physician should also question when the hair was cut last. Frequently cut hair will show less evidence of damage than infrequently cut hair. If the damaged hair shaft ends have been removed prior to visiting the dermatologist, the full extent of hair damage may not be appreciated; however, chemical processing damages the entire hair shaft and problems will reappear shortly.

Is there evidence of heat damage to the hair shaft?

Lastly, the hair should be assessed for heat damage. Heat damage is typically seen as the presence of 'bubble' hair under the electronmicroscope.[8] Bubble hair results from the rapid exposure of the hair shafts to high heat, such as that generated by a curling iron.[9] The water in the hair shaft immediately turns to steam and tries to escape from the hair. This leads to the formation of bubbles within the hair shaft that pop off the cuticular scale. Figure 7.6 shows a hair bubble missing the overlying cuticular scale. However, bubble hair cannot be seen with the naked eye. Visually, hair that has experi-

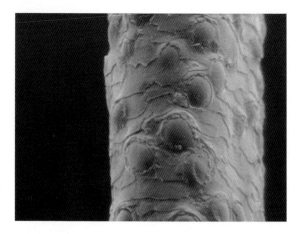

Figure 7.6
An electron micrograph demonstrating bubble hair.

enced heat damage is frizzy with extreme frizziness seen at the ends of the hair shafts due to denaturation of the hair protein. This hair is weak and will readily fracture, even with minimal tension applied by hand. Patients who are experiencing heat damage should be cautioned by the physician to change their hair care practices.

CAUSES OF COSMETIC-INDUCED HAIR LOSS

The prior discussion addressed the mental algorithm to follow to determine if cosmetic-induced hair loss was occurring. This section takes the thought process one step further and presents expanded information on the causes of cosmetic-induced hair loss.

Scalp scratching

Even though mild-to-moderate seborrheic dermatitis does not cause hair loss, the scratching associated with the scalp pruritus can definitely predispose to hair loss. It is possible to remove all of the cuticular scale from a hair shaft with only 90 minutes of continuous scratching by the fingernails. This loss of cuticular scale leaves the hair shaft weakened and permanently cosmetically damaged. Thus, treatment of scalp itch is important in preventing hair loss.

Long vs short hair

Long hair is much more likely to be cosmetically damaged than short hair. Therefore, patients who have extensive hair damage may wish to select a shorter hairstyle to maximize the appearance of the hair. In this case, it is extremely important to identify the cause of the hair damage so that the newly grown hair remains healthy and cosmetically attractive.

Age-related factors

It is a well known fact that hair growth slows down with age. This means that cosmetically damaged hair will be present longer on mature individuals. Also, the diameter of the hair shaft decreases with advancing age. This predisposes the thinner hair shafts to chemical damage from chemical processing. For this reason, all chemicals used on mature hair should be weaker than those used on youthful hair.

Hair combing and brushing

Hair combing is a daily grooming ritual that frequently causes hair damage and loss. Hair should only be combed when dry, if possible. Wet hair is more elastic than dry hair, meaning that vigorous combing of the moist fibers can stretch the shaft to the point of fracture. The ideal comb should be made of a flexible plastic and possess smooth, rounded, coarse teeth that will easily slip through the hair.

Extensive hair brushing should also be avoided while hair is wet. A good brush should have smooth, ball-tipped, coarse, bendable bristles. The brush should not tear the hair, but rather gently glide. Brushes used while blow-drying hair should be vented to prevent increased heat along the brush, which could damage hair. Patients should be encouraged to brush and manipulate their hair as little as possible to minimize breakage. Older teachings that the hair should be brushed 100 strokes a day and the scalp vigorously massaged with the brush should be dispelled.

Hair clasps

Common sense applies to the selection of appropriate hairpins and clasps. Rubber bands should never be used; hairpins should have a smooth, ball-tipped surface; and hair clasps should have spongy rubber padding where they contact the hair. Loose-fitting clasps also minimize breakage. The fact remains, however, that all hairpins or clasps break some hair since they must hold the hair tightly to stay in place. To minimize this problem, the patient should be encouraged to vary the clasp placement so that hair breakage is not localized to one scalp area. This problem is particularly apparent in women who wear a ponytail. These women frequently state that their hair is no longer growing when in actuality it is repeatedly broken at the same distance from the scalp due to hair clasp trauma. Pulling the hair tightly with clasps or braids can also precipitate traction alopecia.

Hair shaft architecture

It is important to remember that curlier hair tends to fracture more readily than straight hair. For this reason, hair shaft architecture can determine how aggressively the hair can be groomed. The kinky hair of African-American patients should be gently groomed with a wide-toothed comb or hair pick. Only Asian hair can be combed with minimal friction and hair shaft damage.

Hair cutting techniques

The hair should always be cut with sharp scissors. Any defect in the scissor blade will crush and damage the hair shaft. Crushing the end of the hair shaft predisposes to split ends.

Hairstyling product use

Hairstyling products are an important way to improve the cosmetic appearance of the hair shaft, but should always leave the hair shaft flexible. High-hold stiff styling products can actually precipitate hair breakage when trying to restyle the hair with combing.

Hairstyling techniques

In general, the less that is done to the hair, the healthier it will be. There is no hairstyle or procedure that can reverse hair damage, even though many salon owners would disagree. Hair is basically a textile. It looks best when new and degrades with age and use.

Hair coloring and bleaching

Hair coloring and bleaching are universally damaging to the hair shaft. It is sometimes said that chemical processing adds body to the hair. This means that the dyeing procedure allows the hair to stand away from the scalp with greater ease. This is not due to better hair health, but rather to hair damage that makes the hair frizzy and more susceptible to static electricity. The basic rule of hair dyeing is: always stay within your color group, preferably dyeing the hair no more than three shades from the natural color.

Hair relaxing

Hair relaxing is weakening to the hair shaft, but can actually facilitate hair length in patients with kinky hair. This is due to decreased hair breakage during combing. The relaxing procedure straightens the hair and makes it easier to groom, but the grooming should be done gently to avoid hair shaft fracture.

Hair permanent waving

Lastly, hair permanent waving is also damaging. The curls should be as loose as possible with the interval between procedures as long as possible. For patients with damaged hair, the perming solution should be weak and left in contact with the hair for as short a period as possible.

TREATMENT OF COSMETIC-INDUCED HAIR LOSS

The treatment of cosmetic-induced hair loss can indeed present a challenge for the physician. This final discussion presents some simple ideas for patients desiring advice in terms of hair cleansing, conditioning, drying, combing, brushing, styling, dyeing and curling.

Hair cleansing

Cleansing the hair should be done only when required due to dirt in the hair or excess sebum. If sebum production is minimal and the patient has a sedentary lifestyle, daily washing is not necessary for good hygiene. The patient should select a shampoo appropriate for their hair type: normal, oily, dry, fine, damaged, or chemically treated. These labels usually appear on the outside of the shampoo bottle. If the patient with normal-to-minimal sebum production insists on daily shampooing, a dry hair shampoo with less detergent action should be recommended. Aggressive removal of sebum results in hair that tangles readily, appears dull, and attracts static electricity.

Hair conditioning

An instant conditioner or a cream rinse can be valuable in minimizing hair loss by detangling the hair, especially long hair.[10] Patients who have excess sebum production may prefer a cream rinse over a conditioner. All formulations of instant conditioners are good at detangling hair by smoothing the cuticle and reducing friction. However, if the hair has been severely damaged and the cuticular scales are sparse with the presence of trichoptilosis, only a protein-containing conditioner can penetrate the hair shaft and temporarily mend split ends.[11] This is due to the substantivity of protein conditioners for hair keratin.

Hair drying

It is best if the hair is allowed to dry without externally applied heat; however, many patients wish to speed up the drying process or style their hair while drying. Heat damage can be avoided by using the lowest heat setting and holding the hairdryer nozzle at least 6 inches from the scalp. A specially designed vented blow-drying brush should be used to prevent high temperatures from reaching the hair along the brush.

Hairstyling

Hairstyling should be done gently on dry hair to minimize breakage. Hairstyles should be loose and not require excessive hairpins or combs. All hairpins should be rubber-coated with smooth edges so that the hair is not broken as the clasp is closed. Rubber bands should not be used in the hair as they are difficult to remove.

Hair appliances

Burning of the hair and subsequent breakage can also be caused by heated hair appliances: curling irons, crimping irons, straightening irons, and heated curlers. Most patients prefer to use these appliances at their hottest setting as this produces the tightest, longest-lasting curl, but it also induces the most hair damage. This burning is minimized if a lower heat setting is chosen. It is also advisable to unplug the heated curlers about 2–3 minutes before placing them in the hair so as to allow slight cooling. Curling, crimping and straightening irons should be placed in a wet towel for a few minutes to allow cooling prior to hair contact.

Hair coloring

In general, darkening the natural hair color is less damaging than lightening the natural hair color, as the original eumelanins and pheomelanins are not removed. Any lightening of the hair color requires the use of hydrogen peroxide to remove existing pigments. In general, the more bleaching required to achieve the final hair color, the weaker the hair shaft at the end of the chemical process. Many patients erroneously think that if bleached blond hair is redyed to their darker original color, it will be healthier. This is not true. Any further dyeing only contributes to additional weakening of the hair shaft.

Hair permanent waving

Permanent waving of the hair is more damaging than dyeing since the protein structure of the hair shaft is actually degraded and reconstructed in a new form. Permanent waving alone decreases hair strength by 15%. Damage can be minimized, however, by wrapping the hair loosely around larger curlers. This results in a looser, shorter-lasting curl, but breakage is minimized.

The processing time can also be shortened, which decreases the degree of bond breaking. The processing time is checked by performing a 'test curl.' The test curl is one rod, usually selected at the nape of neck, where the hair is periodically unwound to determine if the desired amount of curl has been achieved. Not all cosmetologists use a test curl, but it is highly recommended. It is also recommended that the test curl not be placed at the nape of the neck, but rather at the front hairline. Traditionally, the nape of the neck is chosen because this hair is more difficult to permanently wave than any other area of the scalp. If the appropriate amount of curl is present at the nape, then the rest of the scalp will also be curled. However, hair at the front hairline curls more readily and may be overprocessed by the time the nape has curled. This accounts for patients noting more breakage at the anterior hairline.

Many patients both permanently dye and wave their hair. While the damage produced by these procedures is additive, it can be minimized by allowing 10 days between procedures and permanently waving the hair first followed by dyeing the hair.

REFERENCES

1. Wortmann F, Wiesche E, Bourceau B. Analyzing the laser-light reflection from human hair fibers. II. Deriving a measure of hair luster. *J Cosmet Sci* 2004;**55**:81–93.
2. McMullen R, Jachowicz J. Optical properties of hair: effect of treatments on luster as quantified by image analysis. *J Cosmet Sci* 2003;**54**:335–51.
3. Wolfram L, Lindemann MO. Some observations on the hair cuticle. *J Soc Cosmet Chem* 1971;**2**:839.
4. Rook A. The clinical importance of 'weathering' in human hair. *Br J Dermatol* 1976;**95**:111.
5. Robbins C. Weathering in human hair. *Text Res J* 1967;**37**:337.
6. Keis K, Ramaprasad R, Kamath Y. Studies of light scattering from ethnic hair fibers. *J Cosmet Sci* 2004;**55**:49–63.
7. Signori V. Review of the current understanding of the effect of ultraviolet and visible radiation on hair structure and options for photodegradation. *J Cosmet Sci* 2004;**55**: 95–113.

8. Ruetsch S, Kamath Y. Effects of thermal treatments with a curling iron on hair fiber. *J Cosmet Sci* 2004;**55**:13–27.

9. Detwiler SP, Carson JL, Woosley JT et al. Bubble hair. *J Am Acad Dermatol* 1994;**30**:54–60.

10. Menkart J. Damaged hair. *Cutis* 1979;**23**:276–8.

11. Swift J. Mechanism of split-end formation in human head hair. *J Soc Cosmet Chem* 1997;**48**:123–6.

8 Methods for camouflaging hair loss

Occasionally, it is necessary to examine methods for camouflaging hair loss in a patient who may be experiencing hair loss on a permanent or temporary basis. The earlier chapters of this book have examined methods of preserving and beautifying existing hair. This chapter takes a completely different approach to the topic of hair by examining the many excellent options that are available to the patient with thinning or absent hair.

There are a variety of hair prostheses available, including wigs, hairpieces, and toupees, for the individual who still has some remaining scalp hair. For the patient who has lost all scalp hair, vacuum prostheses are discussed as an excellent option. The illusion of abundant hair can be restored through the use of various hair attachment methods including hair braiding, bonding, and fusion for patients with localized hair loss. Lastly, the scalp can be pigmented through the implantation of tattoo pigment to minimize contrast between the white scalp and the darker thinning hair. In all patients, hair cosmetics can be used to increase hair volume. All of these issues are discussed to help the physician counsel the patient with thinning or absent hair.

Before this discussion is undertaken, it is interesting to pause for a moment to examine the rich and colorful history behind wigs and hairpieces. The concept of the wig was originated by the Egyptians in 3000 BC. Many of these elaborate wigs constructed from beeswax-coated vegetable and human hair fibers still survive in museums around the world. These wigs were worn by men and women of the Egyptian ruling class. Blond wigs were worn by the Roman ruling class in the first century BC made of hair taken from German captives, but these blond wigs eventually became the trademark of Roman prostitutes and outlawed by the Christian church. Wigs were rediscovered by the English queens in 1580 who were afflicted by female pattern hair loss. Mary Queen of Scots was never seen without a wig, a fact unknown by her followers until she was beheaded. The popularity of wigs spread from England to France such that the French court of Versailles employed 40 resident wigmakers.[1]

WIGS

Wigs are useful to camouflage hair loss in women with overall scalp hair thinning.

They are formed by attaching individual fibers to a meshwork designed to be worn as a cap over the entire scalp. Two methods of attaching hair fibers to the mesh are used: hand-tied and machine-wefted. Hand-tied wigs are more expensive because the fibers are individually knotted to the mesh. Machine-wefted wigs are made by sewing the fibers onto strips of material and then attaching wefts to the mesh. Friction is required between the cap and the scalp for the wig to remain in place, thus some hair on the head is required to prevent the wig from slipping from side to side.

There are other variations in wig manufacture besides the method used to secure the fibers to the cap. The fibers themselves can be crafted from synthetic sources or from natural human hair fibers. Many persons who are purchasing a wig may think that a human hair wig would provide the most natural appearance, but the synthetic fiber wigs are actually much less expensive and easier to care for than the human hair variety. A custom-made natural human hair wig costs between $1000 and $2000. Typically, the wig is constructed from Asian hair that has been dyed and chemically treated to match the hair appearance of the patient. However, these human hair wigs have a short life of 2–3 years and are prone to experience all of the problems of human hair. This includes hair breakage and the need to restyle the hair on a bi-weekly basis. Synthetic hair products are less expensive, in the range of $100-$1000, and have a longer life of 3–5 years. Synthetic fiber wigs are much easier to maintain. The synthetic fibers have a permanent curl and are much stronger than natural human hair. They also tend to hold their color better and are less prone to environmental factors such as rain, humidity, wind, and sun exposure.

Human hair or synthetic wigs are cleaned in much the same manner as a head of hair. The wig is turned inside out and a drop of mild shampoo is placed in the center and gently agitated under a stream of warm water. Once the shampoo is completely removed, a drop of instant conditioner is placed in the wig and again rinsed. The wig is allowed to air-dry while inside out by attaching it with a clothespin to an indoor clothesline. Once dry, the wig may be styled with a specially designed wig brush. Care should be taken when styling the wig not to break the hair fibers. Typically, a wig will need some repair to either the cap or restoration of damaged fibers on an annual basis. This reconditioning can be done by the wig manufacturer.

The biggest disadvantage to wearing a wig is the warmth and weight of the hairpiece. Many patients in southern climates find the wig hot. Others find the wig heavy and a source of neck strain. It is interesting to note that in general synthetic fiber wigs are lighter than human hair varieties. Wigs may also cause breakage of the patient's remaining hair. This means that patients who wear wigs may notice that their hair is not growing longer since it is being broken by the slight movement of the wig on the head produced with movement.

HAIRPIECES

Hairpieces are designed to cover a localized area of the scalp, whereas a wig is designed to cover the entire scalp. Hairpieces come in a variety of types based on the area and amount of the scalp they are to cover (Table 8.1).

Female patients with localized hair loss on the top of scalp could select a fall or a demiwig to camouflage crown and anterior scalp loss. The demiwig would be for more diffuse loss and the fall for loss primarily at the crown. Toupees would be the analogous

Table 8.1 Types of hairpieces

Hairpiece name	Hairpiece design	Function
Falls	Long locks of hair on woven base	Worn to cover hair loss on scalp vertex
Cascades	Curled locks of hair or a bun attached to a firm base	Worn over the back of the head to create the illusion of hair length
Toupees	Short hair for a male sewn to a silk flexible base	Worn to cover hair loss on the top of the male head
Demiwigs	Flexible cap hairpiece	Designed to cover the entire scalp except the anterior hairline
Wiglets	Small localized hairpiece affixed with hairpins	Designed to add the illusion of bangs or add a small amount of hair on top of the head
Switch	Long strands of hair attached to a woven band	Designed to add the illusion of braids or a ponytail

(a)
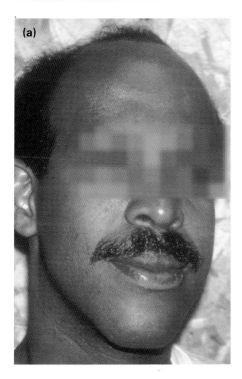

(b)
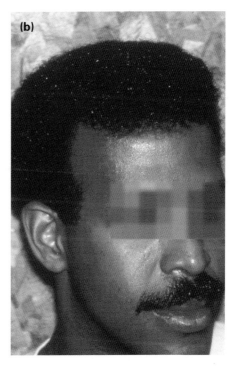

Figure 8.1
Patient before (a) and after (b) application of a toupee to the top of the head.

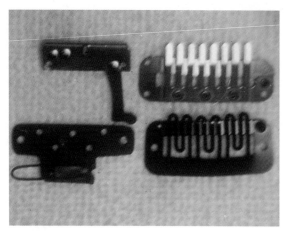

Figure 8.2
Attachment clips used for toupees that can cause hair breakage.

hairpiece for the balding male and are available in a variety of colors with the appropriate percentage of gray hair to match the patient's state of canities (Figure 8.1). Natural part line toupees, which add a small insert of sheer plastic in the part line to expose the natural color of the underlying scalp, may create a more natural appearance. Some toupees come uncut, allowing the patient to take the toupee to the barber for styling along with the patient's natural hair. However, attachment of toupees to the scalp remains poor, relying on clips or adhesives (Figure 8.2). The clips are placed around the periphery of the hairpiece and allow attachment to the remaining scalp hair (Figure 8.3). Unfortunately, the toupee and the attachment clips can result in further hair loss due to breakage and traction alopecia (Figure 8.4).

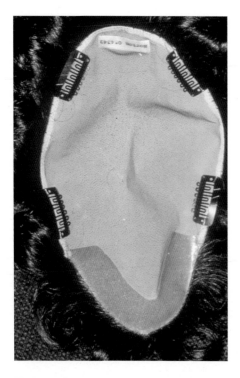

Figure 8.3
Toupee with attachment clips.

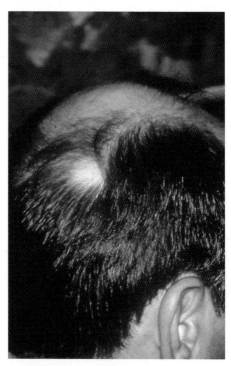

Figure 8.4
Localized hair loss due to hair breakage from use of toupee clips.

There are some hairpieces that can be adapted for patients with special needs. These include cascades designed to camouflage loss on the posterior scalp. Figure 8.5 presents a patient with hair loss caused by radiation treatment for a brain tumor. This patient had a cascade specially designed to allow the patient to pull her existing hair through the hairpiece both to create a more natural appearance and to help anchor the hairpiece (Figure 8.6). Figure 8.7 demonstrates how the patient used a French braid to weave her natural hair in with the hairpiece to create an attractive look. Other special hairpieces known as wiglets can be used to add bangs for a chemotherapy patient who is wearing a turban to camouflage complete hair loss or a switch can be used to add a ponytail or curls for the patient who is regrowing her hair following chemotherapy.

Switches can also be used by African-American women to create the image of abundant curls when the hair is worn short (Figure 8.8).

In closing this discussion, a word should be said about the patient who is anticipating a treatment that will result in temporary or permanent hair loss. It is recommended that these patients select a hairpiece prior to complete hair loss, thus allowing emotional adjustment and a gradual introduction and familiarity with the hairpiece. It is also helpful to have some remaining hair to aid in selecting a wig that mimics the patient's natural hair color and style. If this is not possible, a picture of the patient prior to hair loss should be provided to the wig artist.

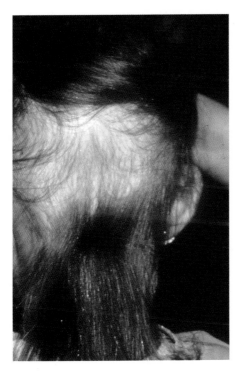

Figure 8.5
Localized hair loss on the posterior scalp.

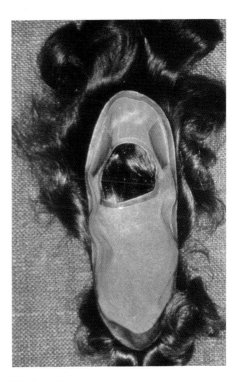

Figure 8.6
Hairpiece specially designed for localized hair loss.

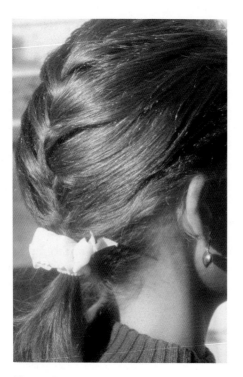

Figure 8.7
Attractive final appearance of
hairpiece on patient.

VACUUM PROSTHESES

These are special hair prostheses designed for individuals with no scalp hair. These patients cannot wear traditional wigs and hairpieces because there is no existing hair to anchor the prostheses. Special prostheses for patients with alopecia totalis or complete permament hair loss due to radiation therapy or other causes are available. These are known as vacuum prostheses, since they rely on the use of a custom-fitted rigid cap that stays in place through the creation of a vacuum between the scalp and the wig. Figure 8.9 illustrates a male patient with long-standing alopecia universalis. His scalp is marked to determine exactly where and how the vacuum prosthesis will fit. A plaster mold is made of his scalp to insure that an

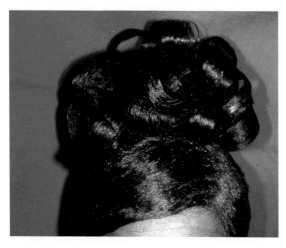

Figure 8.8
A switch of curls on top of the scalp.

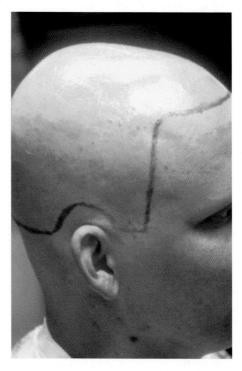

Figure 8.9
Scalp markings to specify wig extent.

exact cast can be made (Figure 8.10). The plaster mold is then turned into an acrylic cap that is fitted prior to the attachment of hair (Figure 8.11). Once the mold has been checked, it is sent back to the wig manufacturer to attach hair of the shape and color of the patient's natural hair, but all of the hair is the same length (Figure 8.12). The patient then goes to his barber with the wig in place and has his hair cut and styled (Figure 8.13). This creates a natural-looking wig that is unique to the patient (Figure 8.14). Before placing the wig on the scalp, the patient applies a gel and then slips on the rigid hairpiece. This creates a vacuum that holds the hair on the scalp until it is firmly pushed to the side for removal. Wigs of this type can provide a natural appearance for patients who have little hope of regrowing their own hair.

Vacuum prostheses represent an option for the patient who has no hair. As might be imagined, they are hot and require some skill for proper attachment. These types of hairpieces are more acceptable in adults than children. They are quite expensive to manufacture and maintain, but can be worn during exercise and most activities, except swimming.

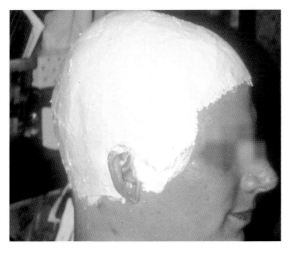

Figure 8.10
Plaster is applied to the scalp to create a cast of the head where the wig will sit.

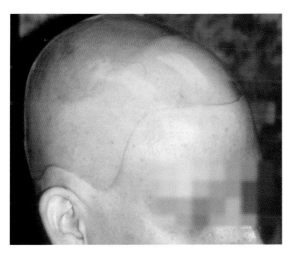

Figure 8.11
The clear acrylic wig base is checked for an accurate fit.

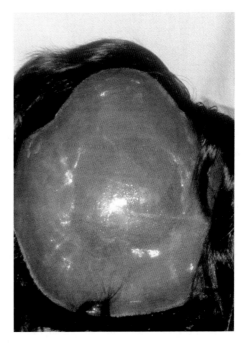

Figure 8.12
The appearance of the finished wig.

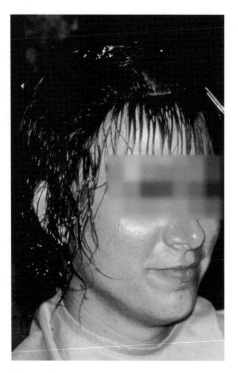

Figure 8.13
Patient having wig trimmed to his
specifications.

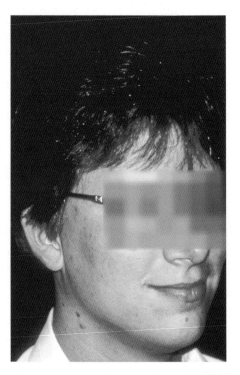

Figure 8.14
Final appearance of vacuum
prosthesis on patient.

HAIR ADDITIONS

Thus far the discussion has focused on wigs
and hairpieces that are worn on a temporary
basis. Most people remove their wigs during
bathing and while sleeping. However,
recently hair additions have become popular
as they are worn continually until they are
redone every 2–8 weeks depending on the
hairstyle. Hair additions utilize synthetic or
natural human hair fibers to supplement
existing hair where needed. The hair fibers
are attached to the scalp or to the existing
hair through a variety of techniques including braiding, bonding, and gluing. Hair additions may be obtained in full service beauty
salons or at salons specializing in the technique. Hair additions are used widely in the
entertainment industry, by African-American
persons who wish to achieve hair length, by
males who wish to camouflage androgenetic alopecia, and by females who desire
special effect hairstyles.

Hair additions involve the use of synthetic
or human hair fibers to enhance the natural
hair. Synthetic fibers are more popular
because they are less expensive and lighter.
Most synthetic hair is formed from
modacrylic, composed of two polymerized
monomers, acrylonitrile and vinylchloride.
The polymer is drawn through a multihole
metal disk, dried and stretched. The disk

design is such that fibers with an irregular cross-section and surface variations are produced to more closely mimic natural human hair. Dye may be added to the polymer either before or after extrusion to produce a multitude of natural and unnatural hair colors. A skilled hair addition artist will take care to mix fibers of varying diameters and color hues, as not all natural hair shafts are of the same thickness or color. The hair addition artist will also select synthetic fibers that mimic the patient's natural African-American, Caucasian, or Oriental hair. The modacrylic is an extremely versatile fiber that can be permanently heat formed to reproduce the appropriate amount and tightness of curl unique to the hair of different ethnic groups.

Rarely, human hair is used for hair additions. This natural hair is obtained from Indian or Chinese women who grow their hair for sale. Indian hair has a fine diameter and a slight natural wave, whereas Chinese hair is coarser and straighter. Usually, the human hair is lightened and redyed to obtain a range of colors and may also be permanently waved to obtain the desired amount of curl. Coloring and curling of hair used in additions may be performed both before and after the added hair is attached to the scalp using standard salon products. Human hair does not require the color and fiber diameter mixing of synthetic hair fibers, as natural variations are already present. Thus, the main advantage of human hair additions is their ability to blend with existing scalp hair. Disadvantages include the weight of the natural fibers and the cost, which increases with longer lengths of hair.

There are a variety of methods that can be used to attach the hair addition to the scalp or to existing hair. These include braiding, bonding, gluing, and lacing, which are discussed next. The method selected depends on the patient's wishes and the amount of hair to be added.

Braiding

The most popular method of hair addition employs braiding. Braiding can be performed either on or off the scalp. Braiding on the scalp involves the use of braids, also known as cornrows, that have been adapted from traditional African hairstyles. Cornrows are plaited on the scalp in geometric designs with tension applied to the hair shafts exposing scalp between the braids. This is a popular hairstyle among Black individuals as it allows for organization of tightly kinked hair. Individual hair fibers can be woven into the braids to either thicken their appearance or, more commonly, to add length. Wefted hair, or hair fibers sewn together in a strip, can be sewn with a needle and thread to the cornrows to add large amounts of hair quickly. Braiding on the scalp can also be used to attach toupees or other hairpieces as shown in Figure 8.15.

Braiding off the scalp employs a standard plaiting technique to which individual hair fibers are added. Fibers are attached by working them securely into the braids and leaving the loose ends for curling and styling. This technique is popular among individuals with short kinky hair who wish to have long straight hair (Figure 8.16). The major problem with braiding off the scalp is traction alopecia (Figure 8.17). The long hair additions are heavy and exert constant traction on the short hairs to which they are attached on the scalp. This traction alopecia is most pronounced around the anterior hair line and can even be observed in young women.

Bonding

Bonding employs a hot glue gun, instead of braiding, to fuse individual synthetic hair fibers to the base of clumps of existing scalp

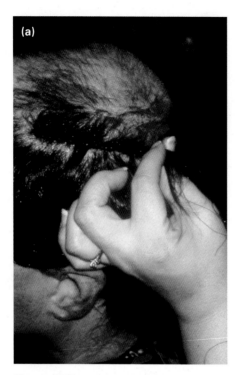
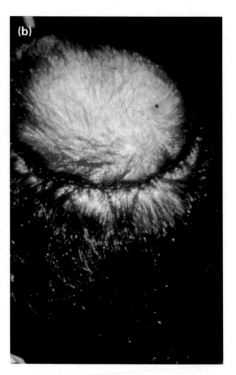

Figure 8.15
(a) A braid is on the scalp to provide (b) an attachment for a toupee to camouflage male pattern baldness.

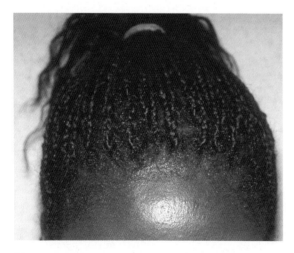

Figure 8.16
Braiding off the scalp to create the illusion of long hair.

hair. Only a few fibers can be attached at a time, due to the weight of the additions. This technique is used in both men and women to thicken the hair. The bonds are intended to remain in place for 8 weeks; however, individuals with excessive sebum production may notice early loosening and loss of the added hair. Bonding is popular in the movie industry to quickly add hair that is intended to be worn for a short period of time.

Gluing

Gluing is similar to bonding, except that large amounts of hair are anchored to the scalp, typically in the form of a modified

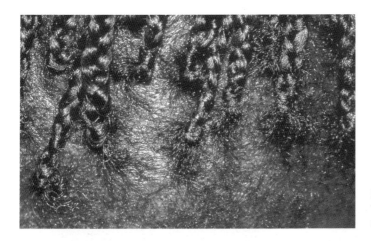

Figure 8.17
Traction alopecia from hair braiding off the scalp.

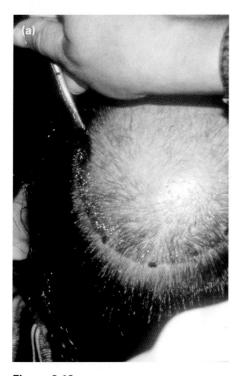

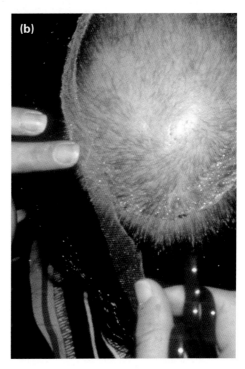

Figure 8.18
(a) The hair has been shaved and glue applied followed by (b) attachment of a woven mesh.

hairpiece. The hair over the area where the hairpiece is to reside is typically shaved or cut close to the scalp. Glue is then applied to facilitate attachment of a woven mesh (Figure 8.18). These tracks serve as anchors to which the hairpiece is glued (Figure 8.19). The adhesive employed is a cold latex-based glue that is subject to removal by scalp

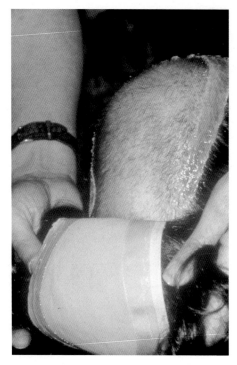

Figure 8.19
The hairpiece is glued to the top of the scalp.

sebum production. Gluing can also be used to attach smaller hair additions to the scalp.

Lacing

Another related technique is hair lacing, also known as hair extensions. Hair lacing involves braiding the patient's natural hair with synthetic or natural hair fibers initially on the scalp and then off the scalp. The braids are stopped 1–2 inches from the scalp and the added hair is allowed to flow freely. The extensions create the illusion of long braided hair and can be woven in many patterns and adorned with beads or jewels. The hairstyle remains in place for 2–8 weeks and is shampooed in place, requiring minimal grooming. The lacing must be completely removed and redone as the hair grows and loosens the hairstyle. Traction alopecia and seborrheic dermatitis are frequently associated with hair extensions, since the added hair is heavy and exerts tension on the scalp, and the infrequent shampooing predisposes to fungal overgrowth.[2]

Care of hair additions

Hair additions are worn continually for a period of 8 weeks, or less, at which time they must be removed. Individuals with slowly growing hair may wear the hairstyle longer, while those with rapidly growing hair notice that the added hair fibers loosen more quickly. The additions are shampooed along with the individual's existing hair using the same cleansing products and cleansing frequency. Many individuals are afraid to wash the additions, concerned that the added hair fibers will loosen, but good hygiene is important.

Removal of hair additions

Hair additions must be removed at 8 weeks to avoid hygiene problems and other complications such as traction alopecia. If the hair and scalp have been properly cleansed, hair additions begin to loosen and look ungroomed at 8 weeks. Removal of the hair additions can be a challenge depending on the attachment technique selected. On the scalp or off the scalp braids are the easiest to remove since the braided additions are simply unbraided and the added strands of hair are undone. These added synthetic or natural hair strands can be reused in subsequent procedures, if desired. However, bonded and glued additions are difficult to remove properly without damaging the patient's own hair. Bonded additions are removed by melting the hot glue with the tip of the glue gun and pulling out the individual or wefted hair fibers. Any remaining glue is loosened and removed by rubbing peanut oil through the scalp. Glued hair additions are usually affixed to the scalp with a latex-based glue that can be loosened with a special solvent. As might be imagined, any bonding or gluing technique results in patient hair loss, making braiding the best method for hair additions.

Patients are sometimes reluctant to have the hair additions removed, but intermittent rest periods are important for the scalp. Ideally, the hair addition should be worn for 8 weeks followed by a 4-week rest period to avoid traction alopecia. It is understandable that patients would like to wear the additions as long as possible, since the style is both expensive and time-consuming. The cost for a hair addition style may vary between $250 and $1000 depending on the complexity of the style, the amount and length of the added hair fibers, the composition of the added hair, and the salon time required. The average hair addition requires 3–5 hours in a salon to style and 1–2 hours to remove.

Adverse effects

Successful use of hair additions requires a hairstylist who is trained in the technique and a patient who will put forth the effort to maintain the added hair. As mentioned previously, braided hair additions pose the least problem as no adhesives are used; however, the added hair fibers put increased pull on existing scalp hair. For this reason, traction alopecia is a common problem in patients who continually wear hair additions. Hair addition traction alopecia is identical to that seen in African-American patients who wear tightly pulled hairstyles. Initially, only loss of the hair shaft is observed, but with continued traction, the process can result in loss of the follicular ostia and permanent alopecia. Extensive traction alopecia will eventually preclude the use of hair additions, as no existing scalp hair will be available to anchor added hair. This information should be shared with patients who are not inclined to remove their hair additions. Failure to remove the additions will eventually require that the patient wear a wig!

The most common side effects are seen with the glued and bonded hair additions. The glues are typically latex-based, which may present a problem for the latex-sensitive patient who may experience allergic contact dermatitis. Also, the removal solvents may be irritating to the scalp, resulting in irritant contact dermatitis. Both allergic and irritant contact dermatitis from the use of hair adhesives are rare, more common problems are related to the actual gluing procedure. If the hairstylist carelessly applies glue throughout the scalp, hair breakage will be increased due to combing problems. Hair additions that require the use of a hot glue gun must also be carefully applied to avoid burning the scalp with either the hot glue or the gun itself. There is no substitute for a well-trained stylist.

Lastly, high standards of hygiene must be maintained to prevent inflammation of the scalp in the form of seborrheic dermatitis and infection. Patients need to understand that the scalp must be kept clean, despite the presence of the added hair. Shampooing is necessary to prevent the growth of fungal and bacterial organisms, even though it may be harder to reach the scalp due to the hair addition. Hair additions require more grooming and upkeep than natural scalp hair.

HAIR INTEGRATION

Hair additions require the attachment of the added hair fibers to existing hair, while hair integration systems attach hair to a fenestrated woven mesh that is worn next to the scalp. The patient's natural hair is pulled through the fenestrations in the mesh to anchor the hair integration system. Hair integration is a useful method for supplementing hair loss only in the necessary areas. These hairpieces are custom-made by fashioning a loose net to fit the scalp. Synthetic or natural human hair fibers are tied to the meshwork in the desired location, amount, length, color and texture (Figure 8.20). Any hairstyle can be created easily. Integration systems can be rather costly depending upon the amount and length of hair

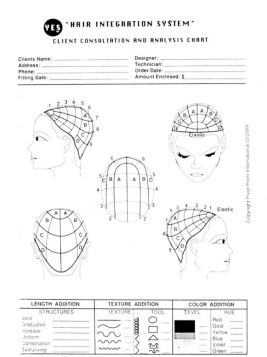

Figure 8.20
A chart used to design a customized hair integration system.

attached. They are extremely versatile for patients with alopecia areata, androgenetic alopecia, scarring alopecia, or radiation-induced hair loss.

SCALP CAMOUFLAGE TECHNIQUES

It is worthwhile briefly mentioning hair loss camouflage techniques that concern the scalp. Often it is the contrast between the pale bald scalp and the dark hair that accentuates hair loss. This contrast can be minimized by temporarily coloring the scalp to match the hair with wax crayons or vegetable dyes. A permanent method of coloring the scalp is with a tattoo. Scalp tattooing is especially helpful for the patient with bitemporal recession and some hair miniaturization. The artistic application of small dots of color can create the illusion of fullness at the anterior hairline, a difficult area to camouflage with a wig or other hairpiece.

HAIR LOSS COSMETIC TECHNIQUES

Hair loss camouflage techniques are most commonly used in women afflicted with female pattern hair loss. This condition begins at puberty with noticeable thinning present by age 40. These women present with hair loss over the entire scalp, but the thinning is most prominent over the fronto-parietal areas with sparing of a thin fringe along the anterior hair line. This pattern was first illustrated by Ludwig.[3] Camouflaging hair loss over the top of the scalp presents a greater challenge than camouflaging hair loss over the sides of the scalp. This means that every attempt should be made to provide appropriate medical treatment for the hair loss before considering cosmetic camouflage methods.[4] This discussion focuses on cosmetic approaches for female and male pattern hair loss in the following areas: hairstyling, hairstyling products, hair permanent waving, and hair coloring agents. The material is presented in a question and answer format to aid the physician in discussing hair loss cosmetic techniques with patients.

What are the best hairstyles for women with female pattern hair loss?

Careful hairstyle selection can minimize the appearance of female pattern hair loss. Since the hair is thinned predominantly on the top of the head, styling techniques should be aimed at adding volume and fullness in this area. The perception of thick hair is based on the distance that the hair stands away from the scalp, but appropriate hairstyling can create the illusion of fullness. Two styling techniques are valuable for creating the illusion of hair volume: curling and backcombing.

How should the hair be curled to create the illusion of hair fullness?

Curled hair does not lie as close to the scalp as straight hair and therefore appears fuller. This is a valuable styling technique in the patient with thinning hair. Temporary curls can be created by heat styling with a blow-dryer and a round brush, setting wet hair on rollers, wrapping hair around heated rollers, or an electric curling rod. Tighter curls will yield more hair fullness. The size of the curl is determined by the diameter of the curling device, with smaller diameter devices yielding tighter curls.

How should the hair be combed to maximize hair volume?

Backcombing is a safe method for maximizing hair volume. This technique involves combing the hair in the opposite direction from which it would normally lie on the scalp. In most females, the hair pattern is such that the hair on the top of the scalp lies forward. Combing the hair backward from the front of the head to the crown lifts the hair, creating the illusion of volume. The hair will not stay in this unnatural position for long, therefore styling aids are necessary for the hair to hold this shape.

What hairstyling techniques should be avoided in patients with female pattern hair loss?

A common technique for increasing hair volume, especially among mature women, is teasing. This damaging hairstyling technique became popular in the 1960s to create the 'beehive' hairstyles. Teasing involves combing the hair from the distal to proximal hair shaft using a fine-toothed comb or teasing brush to create tangles between the hair shafts. These tangles, or 'rats' as they are known, allow the hair to stand away from the scalp. Teasing, however, can result in disruption of the hair shaft cuticle and can accelerate hair breakage. It is important to avoid hair breakage in areas where the hair is already thinned. For this reason, teasing should be avoided in patients with female pattern hair loss. While it is a quick method of achieving hair fullness, ultimately it will result in accelerated hair breakage and loss. A better method of getting the hair to stand away from the scalp and create volume is through the use of the newer hairstyling products.

Which hairstyling products are recommended in the patient with female pattern hair loss?

Hairstyling products are valuable in the female pattern hair loss patient to aid in creating the illusion of fullness by allowing the hair to stand away from the scalp. Available styling products include: styling gels, sculpturing gels, mousses, and hair-sprays. Styling gels, sculpturing gels, and mousses are generally applied to towel-dried hair while hairsprays are used to improve the hold of a finished hairstyle. Sculpturing gels provide stiffer hold than styling gels, which provide better hold than mousses.

How should the styling product be applied to create hair volume?
The styling product application technique is the key to create hair volume. A small amount of gel or mousse is massaged into the base of the hair shafts by the scalp. The hair is then dried with the head upside down by a hand-held blow-dryer set on low fan speed and low heat held about 8 inches from the hair. The hair is combed with the fingers away from the scalp during the drying process. This procedure encourages the hair to set in a position away from the scalp, cre-ating the illusion of volume. Once the hair is dry, it will maintain its shape until rewetted. The hair can be styled as usual.

Can the hair be air-dried and still achieve volume with thinning hair?
A technique known as 'scrunching' can be used to create hair fullness while allowing the hair to air-dry. Sculpturing gel is applied generously to the scalp and proximal hair shafts with a small amount applied to the distal hair shafts. The hair is then sectioned and randomly mashed into 1-inch clumps that are affixed with a hair clip and allowed to air-dry. This will create random waves in the hair that will also create the illusion of fullness. This styling technique can be used to set the hair overnight while sleeping.

Which hairspray is best for male and female patients with thinning hair?
Hairspray is probably the most important styling product for the male or female patient with thinning hair. It is used to keep the final hairstyle in place. For example, after backcombing the hair, it can be liberally sprayed to allow the hair to fall backward instead of forward on the forehead, creating the illusion of volume. Hairspray can also be used to keep the hair in place over thin areas of the scalp.

The best hairsprays are the newer flexible polymer hairsprays that allow the hair to move while keeping the desired style. These hairsprays will say 'flexible' on the label. They prevent hair breakage by allowing the patient to comb and style the hair without tearing the individual hair shafts stiffened by hairspray. Flexible hairsprays can also be combed out of the hair and restyled without the need to shampoo.

Can a person with thinning hair undergo a permanent wave procedure?
Permanent waving is a safe and advisable procedure for the patient with thinning hair if performed properly. Permanent waving increases apparent hair volume through the addition of curls, allowing less hair to cover more scalp. Thus, a permanent wave in the frontoparietal area can nicely camouflage female pattern hair loss. However, chemical curling damages the hair shaft by decreas-ing its strength, degrading its structure, and causing protein loss. This damage can be minimized if the permanent wave is per-formed using a mild perming solution to create a body wave instead of tight pin curls.

How can hair damage be avoided with a permanent wave procedure in a patient with thinning hair?
Hair shaft damage can be decreased with a permanent wave procedure in a patient with thinning hair by following a few simple pointers. First, the hair should be wrapped with minimal tension around the mandrels to prevent hair shaft weakening. Second, larger mandrels should be selected to create

a looser curl. Third, a shorter processing time should be used since the fine thinning hair will process more rapidly. Lastly, it is advisable to allow as much time as possible between permanent waving procedures to minimize hair damage. Persons with thinning hair can successfully undergo a permanent waving procedure provided that these guidelines are followed.

Can hair dyeing be used in male and female patients with thin hair?

Hair color lightening can be an effective camouflage technique for hair loss by providing better blending with a lightly colored scalp. Of all the hair coloring types available, only permanent hair dyes can achieve color lightening, but permanent hair dyes are also the most damaging to the hair shaft. Thus, the hair should be lightened minimally, just enough to minimize the contrast.

REFERENCES

1. Panati C. Atop the vanity. In: *Extraordinary origins of everyday things*. New York: Harper & Row, 1987:234–6.
2. Harman RRM. Traction alopecia due to hair extension. *Br J Dermatol* 1972;**87**:79–80.
3. Ludwig E. Classification of the types of androgenetic alopecia (common baldness) occurring in the female sex. *Br J Dermatol* 1977;**97**:247–54.
4. Bergfeld WF. Etiology and diagnosis of androgenetic alopecia. In: De Villez RL, ed. *Clinics in dermatology* Philadelphia: JB Lippincott, 1988:102–7.

9   Nonlaser hair removal techniques

It always seems that hair grows abundantly where it is not wanted and will not grow where desired. This is the dilemma of many dermatologists who are confronted with the male patient who desires more scalp hair, but wishes to eliminate his ear hair or the female patient who wants treatment for thinning scalp hair, while inquiring about decreasing her arm hair at the same visit. Hair growth is as big a challenge as hair removal. The previous two chapters have dealt with minimizing and camouflaging scalp hair loss. This chapter deals with minimizing hair growth on other body areas. It covers the techniques of wet shaving, dry shaving, plucking, waxing, depilatories, and electrolysis. It does not cover laser hair removal, since this is felt to be a discussion topic for an entire book. This chapter will deal with those techniques that are performed at home or in a hair salon not requiring the supervision of a physician.

It is important to recognize that no single method of hair removal is appropriate for all body locations. This means that the physician must understand all methods for home and salon hair removal, since each has certain inherent strengths and weaknesses (Table 9.1).

WET SHAVING

Wet shaving is the most widespread method of hair removal used today. This is due to the fact that the hair can be rapidly removed very close to the skin surface. It is relatively inexpensive, requiring only the use of a razor and shaving cream. Wet shaving is commonly used by men to remove facial hair and by women to remove armpit, leg, and groin hair. The major drawbacks of wet shaving include irritation of the perifollicular skin, a condition commonly known as razor burn, and the rapidity with which regrowth occurs. This is due to cutting of the hair shafts flush with the skin surface under optimal shaving conditions. Wet shaving produces hairs with sharp edges due to the perpendicular nature of the cut (Figure 9.1). Hair that has never been cut has a naturally tapered soft tip, while wet shaving creates hairs with a bristly feel.[1,2]

The most important part of wet shaving is selection of a quality razor and ancillary shaving products used in the proper fashion. Box 9.1 presents ideas for minimizing skin irritation in patients who are experiencing difficulty with wet shaving. In general, razor designs with an angle of 28–32 degrees between the blade and the skin produce the

Table 9.1 Methods of hair removal

Technique	Equipment	Regrowth period	Body sites for use	Advantages	Disadvantages
Wet shaving	Razor	Days	Face, arms, legs, axilla, groin	Fast, easy, close shave	Razor burn, rapid regrowth
Dry shaving	Electric shaver	Days	Face, arms, legs, axilla	Fast, easy	Poor shave, folliculitis, rapid regrowth
Plucking	Tweezers	Weeks	Eyebrows, facial hair	Slower regrowth	Painful, slow
Waxing	Wax and melting pot	Weeks	Face, eyebrows, groin	Longer regrowth period	Painful slow, skill required
Depilatories	Depilatory	Days	Legs, groin	Quick	Irritating, poor quality hair removal
Electrolysis	Professional operator and equipment	May be permanent	All	May be permanent	Painful time-consuming, expensive

closest shave with the least amount of irritation.[3] There are other factors, however, that the physician can address with the patient who is having shaving-related dermatoses (Box 9.2). Advise all patients to always use a sharp blade. This means that razors should not be stored in the shower. They should be

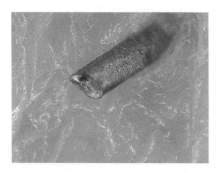

Figure 9.1
End of razor cut hair viewed with a video microscope.

kept in a dry environment where they will not be bumped or damaged. If the razor is accidentally dropped, the blade should be replaced immediately, since it is no longer sharp. It is important to remember that the quality of the shave is based on the worst part of the blade. Any small irregularity in the blade edge will be problematic. The blade should always be sharp, requiring that a blade only be used for three or four shaves, especially if the beard is coarse. Additionally, the razor should not be shared with other individuals. Not only does this spread viral and bacterial infections, but each person shaves differently, thus dulling the blade in a different fashion.

The razor blade design is only part of the shaving equation, however. Equally important is the use of shaving cream. The purpose of shaving cream is to reduce friction between the razor and the skin while soften-

Box 9.1 Methods for minimizing shaving irritation in men and women

1. Select a razor with a handle that fits comfortably in the patient's hand.
2. Use a razor that has replaceable blades. Avoid disposable razors.
3. Spring-mounted, laser-sharpened, triple-bladed razor cartridges work the best (Mach 3 razor, Gillette for men, Venus razor, Gillette for women).
4. Wet the skin with warm water.
5. Apply a post-foaming shaving gel (Edge Gel for Sensitive Skin, SC Johnson).
6. Allow the shaving gel to remain on the skin as a foam for 3–4 minutes.
7. Begin shaving by allowing the razor to glide over the skin with minimal pressure and smooth even strokes.
8. Frequently rinse blade of debris.
9. Never shave over the same area twice.
10. Avoid stretching the skin while shaving.

Box 9.2 Pointers for achieving an optimal shave

1. Never use any razor blade more than four times, especially with a thick beard.
2. If the razor is dropped, replace the blade immediately. It has been damaged.
3. Keep the razor blade perfectly parallel to the skin surface. It has been designed with the optimal shaving angle in mind.
4. Use a shaving cream with a rich, thick lather.
5. Shave in the direction of hair growth. Shaving against the direction of hair growth will increase irritation, but also increase shave closeness.
6. Do not press firmly with the blade against the skin. Allow the razor to glide freely.

ing the hair. The shaving cream softens the hair by increasing water entry into the hair shaft and making it more elastic. This water entry into the hair shaft does not occur immediately. It takes about 3–4 minutes. It is for this reason that the area to be shaved should be wetted with warm water, the shaving cream applied, and allowed to set for 3–4 minutes before shaving. This is the most common mistake made by patients who are experiencing undue folliculitis or razor burn from shaving. The best shaving creams are actually known as post-foaming shave gels. These products soften the beard, lubricate the skin, and reduce razor drag optimally.[4]

Other factors influence the closeness of a shave, which results from the optimum interaction between the blade and the skin. Resilient skin with abundant subcutaneous fat is the best for achieving a close shave with few cuts. This may explain why shaving becomes more of a challenge for mature men with redundant skin and little subcutaneous fat. A smooth skin surface with the absence of deep pits around hair ostia also allows the blade to glide more easily with minimal nicks. This explains why some men have more difficulty achieving a close shave than others. Lastly, men with multiple hairs exiting from one follicular ostia also have difficulty.[3] Thus, genetic factors play a role in determining shaving ease in various patients.

It is also important to allow the blade to do the cutting freely. This means that the blade should be allowed to glide over the skin surface with minimal friction and minimal shaving pressure. Holding the blade at an angle leads to a large shaving angle and a poor quality shave. Excess pressure will cut proportionately more skin and hair. When evaluating a new razor blade design, all the hair and skin removed during the shaving process is collected. The ratio of the hair to skin removed is calculated. If this ratio is low, the blade design is poor. Many patients try to increase the closeness of the shave by shaving against the direction of hair growth. While this will lead to a closer shave, it will also remove proportionately more skin. Repeat shaving over a given area should also be avoided.[5]

The main advantage of wet shaving is that it allows the hair to be cut closely at the skin surface. It is an excellent hair removal technique for large, well-keratinized body surfaces, such as the legs in women and the face of men, where rapid regrowth and a coarse skin texture are not a problem. Females who have keratosis pilaris on the upper outer thighs should use wet shaving over dry shaving as shaving cream can soften the perifollicular keratotic material, thus minimizing skin trauma.

Problems with wet shaving include skin irritation, skin trauma, and the chance of spreading skin infections (such as impetigo or viral verruca) through microscopic tears in the stratum corneum. The regrown hair shafts also have a sharp tip which may reenter the skin resulting in pseudofolliculitis barbae, commonly seen in the neck area of Black patients[6,7] (Figure 9.2).

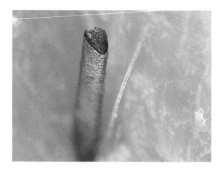

Figure 9.2
Two days' hair growth demonstrating the rough edges of the cut hair.

DRY SHAVING

Dry shaving uses an electric shaver without moisture or shaving cream. The electric shaver contains blades which rotate or vibrate, thereby cutting the hair shaft. In general, an electric shaver cannot cut the hairs as closely to the skin surface as a razor, but skin abrasion is not as great a problem. Skin irritation and the spread of cutaneous infections may still occur.[8] This can be minimized by professionally cleaning and sharpening the shaver every 3 months. It is not unusual for a patient to use a shaver for years without sharpening the blades or removing skin and hair debris.

The advantages of dry shaving include the rapidity and ease with which the hair can be removed. Large surface areas can be shaved with minimal effort, as long as the hair shafts are short. Clippers, a variant of the electric razor, can be used to easily shave longer hairs. The major disadvantage is the inability to achieve a close shave.

In areas where rapid hair regrowth or bristly hair is a problem, such as the face of women, dry shaving should not be used. Furthermore, the sharp regrowing hair shafts may cause irritation in intertrigenous areas such as the underarms or inguinal folds. Dry shaving may also cause irritation of the follicular ostia resulting in perifollicular pustules, a problem seen especially in the female pubic area. In these instances, other methods of hair removal are recommended. Box 9.3 presents tips for achieving the optimal dry shave.

PLUCKING

Plucking of the hair is a method of removing the entire hair shaft, including the bulb, with a pair of tweezers.[9] It is an easy, inexpensive method of hair removal requiring minimal equipment, but can be tedious and mildly uncomfortable. Many patients mistakenly believe that plucking encourages hair growth. This is not the case. The time to regrowth depends upon whether the hair was extracted by the root or broken off at the skin surface. Hairs that are broken at the surface will regrow rapidly, as expected. The proper method for plucking a hair is presented in Box 9.4.

The main disadvantage of plucking is that removal of hair from large areas is not feasible. Plucking is effective for removal of stray eyebrow hairs or isolated coarse hairs on the chin of postmenopausal women, but the

---

Box 9.3 Tips for achieving the optimal dry shave

1. Apply a facial disinfectant prior to shaving, if perifollicular pustules are a frequent problem. Rubbing alcohol or prescription topical clindamycin can be used.
2. Do not press too hard with the shaver.
3. Keep the shaver head clean of hair and skin debris.
4. Sharpen the shaver blades every 3–6 months to prevent the shaver from tearing the hair shafts and damaging the skin. Every 3 months is recommended if the beard hair is coarse.
5. If regrowth is rapid, shave morning and evening with gentle pressure, rather than applying firm pressure to achieve a close shave once daily.

Box 9.4 Proper hair plucking method

1. Select a quality pair of angled tweezers. Look at the tweezers carefully to insure that the tips meet across the entire plucking surface.
2. Select a quality lighted magnification mirror that can stand on a countertop. Place the mirror at eye level.
3. Hold the tweezers in the dominant hand and hold the skin of the area to be plucked tightly in the nondominant hand.
4. Use the angled tip of the tweezers to grasp the hair firmly.
5. Pull the hair with gentle firm pressure until it is removed from the follicular ostia. Do not yank or jerk.
6. Apply a rubbing alcohol swab to the plucked area to minimize post-plucking papules and pustules.

numerous hairs present in the armpits or legs of a female cannot be plucked efficiently. It is also important to remember that only terminal hairs can be plucked efficiently, since vellus hairs usually break close to the skin surface.

One problem with plucking hairs, especially in the eyebrow area, is failure of the hair to regrow after plucking. Generally this would not be thought to be a problem, but the eyebrow hairs in the female decrease in number with age. This means that young women who overpluck their eyebrows may experience almost complete loss of the eyebrows with maturity.[10] Hair transplantation in the eyebrow area remains problematic, meaning that young women should be encouraged not to follow fashion whims requiring pencil-thin eyebrows.

WAXING

Waxing is a variation of hair plucking that is accomplished in a more efficient manner to allow hair removal over a larger body surface area. Two waxing techniques are available: hot waxing and cold waxing. As the names imply, hot waxing involves the application of warm wax to the hair removal area and cold waxing involves the use of a polymer applied at room temperature for hair removal.

Hot waxing is commonly performed in salons to remove unwanted hair from the eyebrows, lateral face, upper lip, and bikini area. It is used for removal of hair on the legs less commonly. Professional hot wax is composed of rosin, beeswax, paraffin wax, petrolatum, and mineral or vegetable oil with or without the addition of menthol. The menthol is sometimes added to create a pleasing smell or to minimize the discomfort associated with hair waxing. The wax is melted in a professional wax pot and carefully applied to the hairs with a wooden spatula (Figure 9.3). The hairs are embedded in the wax, which is allowed to cool and harden. Once the wax has hardened, it is pulled from the skin surface with the hands or with tweezers. The hope is to remove the hair from the follicular ostia at the level of the hair bulb to prolong regrowth. The biggest problem is burning the skin with excessively hot wax.

Cold waxing, a newer hair removal method, employs a wax-like substance that is squeezed as a liquid from a pouch, thus eliminating the need for melting. It is composed of a polymer that hardens to a flexible film at room temperature. Sometimes the polymer is combined with a piece of loosely woven cheese cloth. The cloth is applied to the skin first, followed by the application of the polymer. The loose cloth weave allows the polymer to penetrate through the cloth to the hairs. The cloth is then pulled to remove the wax and the embedded hairs from the skin. The main advantage of the cloth is that it provides strength so the wax can theoretically be removed in one piece rather than numerous smaller pieces (Figure 9.4). Cold waxing, as described in Box 9.5, is the recommended wax removal method for inexperienced home users.

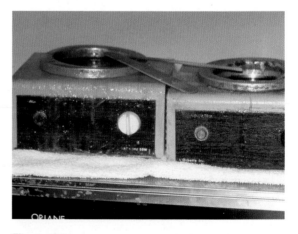

Figure 9.3
Professional wax pot.

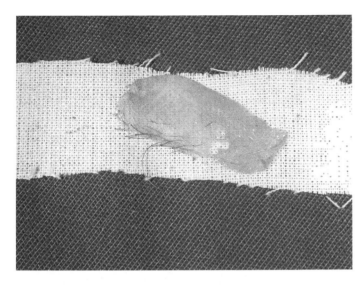

Figure 9.4
A cloth and wax combination that is used for eyebrow waxing.

Box 9.5 Cold wax home hair removal method

1. Wash the skin and the hair thoroughly in the area to be waxed.
2. Be sure that the hair is at least one-sixteenth of an inch long.
3. Apply the cheese cloth over the clean, dry skin surface. Be sure the cloth is in complete contact with the skin with no folds or air spaces.
4. Open the cold wax pouch.
5. Quickly spread the material thinly and evenly over the cheese cloth with the wooden applicator, taking care to insure that the material penetrates the cloth and is in direct contact with the skin.
6. Remain immobile while the material is hardening.
7. Once the material is no longer sticky, gently loosen the edges of the cheese cloth.
8. Pull with firm even tension to remove the cloth, material, and hair from the skin surface. Do not yank, or the hair will be broken at the skin surface and not by the root.
9. Apply a thin layer of petroleum jelly to the skin surface where the hair has been removed to improve barrier function and minimize irritation.

Waxing has the advantage of adequate removal of both terminal and vellus hairs. This is important on the upper lip, chin, eyebrows, cheeks, and groin of women where removal of all hair is desirable. Men generally do not find waxing of facial hair acceptable as the hair has to grow to at least one-sixteenth of an inch before it can be removed reliably by waxing. Excess hair present in Becker's nevi, congenital hairy nevi, and benign hairy nevi can be safely removed in both males and females with the waxing technique.

The major disadvantages of waxing are discomfort and poor removal of hairs shorter than one-sixteenth of an inch.

Patients may also need to tweeze a few hairs that were not removed and thick hair growth may require two treatments for complete removal.

The results of waxing are identical to hair plucking. The 2-week regrowth period is longer than that for shaving, since most of the hairs are removed by the root. When regrowth occurs, the hair has a tapered tip rather than the sharp, blunt tip produced by shaving. No damage to the surrounding skin occurs, but patients must test the heated wax prior to application to avoid a burn. Waxing can be done professionally in a salon or at home. Professional fees vary depending on the size of the removal area. For example, it costs about $20 to have the eyebrows professionally waxed. Home waxing is much less expensive: $4 will purchase sufficient wax to remove excess eyebrow hair for 30 treatments.

DEPILATORIES

Chemical depilatories are similar to shaving in that the hair is removed at the skin surface, except that shaving removes the hair physically and depilatories remove the hair chemically. Depilatories function by softening the hair shaft above the skin surface so it can be gently wiped away with a soft cloth. Presently marketed chemical depilatories are available in pastes, powders, creams and lotions with formulations specially adapted for use on the legs, groin area, and face. All formulations function by softening the cysteine-rich hair disulfide bonds to the point of dissolution. This is accomplished by combining five different classes of ingredients.

The agents combined to produce a chemical depilatory are detergents, hair shaft swelling agents, adhesives, pH adjusters and bond-breaking agents.[11] Together they function to prepare the hair for removal. Detergents such as sodium lauryl sulfate, laureth-23, or laureth-4 remove protective hair sebum and allow penetration of the bond-breaking agent. Further penetration is accomplished with swelling agents such as urea or thiourea. Adhesives such as paraffin allow the mixture to adhere to the hairs while adjustment of pH to 9.0–12.5 minimizes cutaneous irritation. Lastly, the bond-breaking agent is able to successfully destroy the hair shaft.

Several bond-breaking agents are available: thioglycolic acid, calcium thioglycolate, strontium sulfide, calcium sulfide, sodium hydroxide, and potassium hydroxide. The most popular commercial bond-breaking agents are the thioglycolates, as they minimize cutaneous irritation while effectively breaking disulfide bonds; however, they are less effective at dissolving coarse hair such as the male beard. Sulfide bond-breaking agents are faster-acting, but are more irritating and sometimes produce an undesirable sulfur odor. Sodium hydroxide, also known as lye, is the best bond-breaking agent, but is extremely damaging to the skin. These are the same chemicals that are used in hair permanent waving and straightening procedures, except that the chemical reaction is allowed to completely destroy the hair shaft rather than merely inducing bond rearrangement.

Chemical depilatories are applied as a thin layer on the hair-bearing skin for 5–10 minutes. During that time, the hair disulfide bonds are completely broken such that the hair assumes a corkscrew appearance and becomes gelatinous. The hair is wiped away from the skin surface with minimal pressure. As might be expected, shorter fine hair takes less time to respond to the depilatory than coarse long hair. Depilatories are somewhat selective for hair shaft damage, since the hair shaft contains more cysteine than the surrounding skin, but skin irritation can still occur with prolonged contact. Under no circumstances should chemical depilatories be applied to abraded or dermatitic skin. Box 9.6 summarizes these steps in a list for patient use.

Chemical depilatories are best used for removal of hair on the legs of women. Darkly pigmented hair seems somewhat more resistant to removal than lighter hair and coarse hair is more resistant than fine hair. This explains why these products are difficult to use on the male beard. However, a variety of powder depilatories, containing barium sulfide, are available for the Black male who has difficulty with pseudofolliculitis barbae[12,13] (Figure 9.5). These powdered products are mixed with water to form a paste and applied to the beard with a wooden applicator for 3–7 minutes. The hair and depilatory are then removed with the same applicator and the skin is rinsed with cool water. This procedure should be performed no more frequently than every other day.

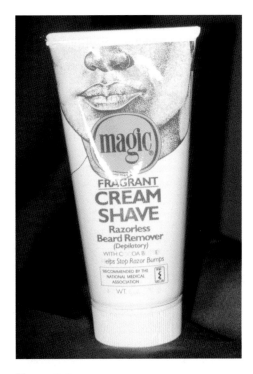

Figure 9.5
A male facial depilatory.

Box 9.6 Depilatory hair removal technique

1. Thoroughly wash the area for depilatory application, removing all sebum and moisturizers. Any oils on the hair will prevent depilatory penetration into the hair shafts.
2. Select a shower or a bathtub for depilatory application, since the procedure is messy and can damage cloth and wood surfaces. The depilatory will also create a sulfur odor during the processing due to the release of sulfur from the disulfide hair bonds.
3. Apply the depilatory in a thin layer to the dry skin and hair.
4. Allow the depilatory to remain on the skin until the hairs have assumed a corkscrew configuration.
5. Check a small area to see if the hair can be easily wiped away with a soft clean old washcloth.
6. If the hair has been adequately softened, wipe all the hair away from the legs.
7. Cleanse the area with a gentle cleanser.
8. Apply a thin layer of petroleum jelly to restore the barrier function and minimize skin irritation.

The main advantage of chemical depilatory hair removal as compared with shaving is the absence of skin cuts, but the major disadvantage is skin irritancy. A study by Richards *et al.* found that fewer than 1% of their female study population could tolerate facial depilatories.[9] Allergic contact dermatitis is less common than irritant contact dermatitis but may be seen due to fragrances, lanolin derivatives, or other cosmetic additives. Generally, depilatories are not appropriate for any patient with dermatologic problems.

ELECTROLYSIS

All of the other hair removal methods discussed thus far have been temporary. There are only two permanent methods of hair removal, electrolysis and laser. Laser hair removal is not discussed in this text, since it must be performed under the direction of a physician. Electrolysis is discussed in detail, since it falls in the realm of cosmetology, the main focus of this text. Electrolysis remains a tremendously popular hair removal technique among women for unwanted hair on the face, chin, neck, and bikini area.[14] Its popularity has endured because it is less expensive than laser hair removal, can be used on all colors of hair and skin, and does not produce permanent skin dyspigmentation. There are three electrolysis techniques: galvanic electrolysis, thermolysis, and the blend.

The first individual to use electrolysis for hair removal was Missouri ophthalmologist Dr Charles E. Michel who used the technique in the treatment of trichiasis in 1875. The technique became popularized during the later part of the nineteenth century. In 1924, the technique of thermolysis was developed by Dr Henri Bordier of Lyon, France. The combination of electrolysis and thermolysis, known as the blend, was developed by Arthur Hinkel and Henri St Pierre in 1945 and a patent was granted for the technique in 1948.[15]

All electrolysis techniques involve the insertion of a needle into the follicular ostia down to the follicular germinative cells (Figure 9.6). The dermal papillae must be destroyed to permanently prevent hair growth. Only hairs that are visible can be removed by electrolysis, and only anagen hairs can be adequately treated. Similar to

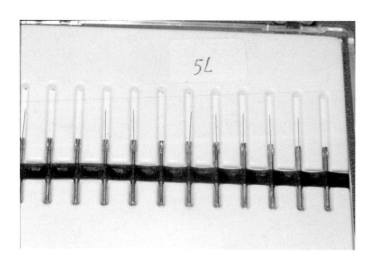

Figure 9.6
An electrolysis needle.

laser hair removal, follicles in the telogen phase without a visible hair shaft cannot be treated. If there is a high telogen to anagen ratio, a substantial amount of hair growth will be seen in the treated area. This ratio varies depending on body area.[16]

Electrolysis is based on heating the water in the hair follicle to a temperature sufficient to destroy the germinative cells of the hair follicle. Water is necessary to transmit the electrical energy between the electrolysis needle and the dermal papillae. Since the lower part of the hair follicle is better hydrated than the more superficial follicle, the electrolysis needle must be inserted to the proper depth. The depth of needle insertion is determined by the hair shaft diameter. As demonstrated in Table 9.2, larger diameter hairs require deeper needle insertion for adequate destruction. Knowledge of follicular depth is necessary to ensure adequate follicular destruction without scarring.

The permanence of the hair removal depends on the degree of damage to the dermal papillae, which is determined by the intensity and duration of the current administered. High intensity energy may be used for a short duration or lower intensity energy may be used for a longer duration. The decision as to how much energy to use depends upon both the technique used by the electrologist and the pain tolerance of the patient. As might be expected, pain increases with higher intensity energy. Low intensity energy, however, is unable to destroy some hairs. In general, coarse hairs require longer treatment duration than fine hairs.[17] Electrolysis is much more difficult to perform on individuals with curly, wavy, or kinky hair. This is due to difficulty in placing the needle accurately into the hair follicle.

Electrolysis, thermolysis, and the blend represent the three techniques that can be used to permanently remove unwanted hair with electricity.[18] Each technique is discussed in detail next.

Electrolysis

The complete name for electrolysis is 'galvanic electrolysis,' so named because it utilizes direct current (DC) which is passed through a stainless steel needle into the tissue sodium chloride and water surrounding the hair follicle. The DC current causes ionization of the salt (NaCl) and water (H_2O) into free sodium (Na+), chloride (Cl−), hydrogen (H+), and hydroxide (OH−) ions. These free ions then recombine into sodium hydroxide (NaOH), also known as lye, and hydrogen gas (H_2). The caustic sodium hydroxide destroys the hair follicle while the hydrogen gas escapes into the atmosphere. The amount of sodium hydroxide produced is greater at the base of the hair follicle due to increased moisture content requiring electrolysis needle insertion deep into the follicle. The amount of follicular destruction induced is measured in units of lye as the amount of lye produced when 0.1 milliamp of current flows for one second.[19] Galvanic

Table 9.2 Hair shaft diameter and hair follicle depth

Hair shaft diameter (inches)	Description of hair	Hair follicle depth (mm)
< 0.001	Very fine	< 1
0.001–0.002	Fine	1–2
0.002–0.003	Medium	2–3
0.003–0.004	Coarse	3–4
0.004–0.005	Very coarse	4–5
0.005–0.006	Extra coarse	5
> 0.006	Super coarse	5

Adapted from Richards RN, Meharg GE. *Cosmetic and medical electrolysis and temporary hair removal.* Ontario: Medric Ltd, 1991.

electrolysis is the most effective method of producing permanent hair removal, but is tedious and slow. This has led to the development of multiple needle techniques where numerous hair follicles can be treated simultaneously.

Thermolysis

Thermolysis, also known as short-wave radio frequency diathermy, differs from galvanic electrolysis in that alternating high frequency (AC) current is passed down the needle. This current causes vibration of the water molecules around the hair follicle and produces heat in a manner similar to a microwave oven.[20] The needle begins to heat at the tip first and spreads toward the skin surface. This means that the heat remains longer around the hair follicle than at the skin surface, minimizing discomfort and cutaneous damage. If too much AC current is administered, steam is produced which exits through the follicular ostia resulting in a burn and possible scarring. Thermolysis is much faster than galvanic electrolysis, but does not destroy the hair follicle as reliably. It is unable to reliably destroy distorted or curved hair follicles.

Blend

The blend is a combination of both galvanic electrolysis and thermolysis.[21] Both direct and high frequency alternating current are passed down the needle at the same time to produce sodium hydroxide and heat. The hot lye is extremely effective at destroying the dermal papillae, allowing superior results with less regrowth. Furthermore, the tissue damage induced by the thermolysis allows the lye to spread through the hair fol-

licle more rapidly. The blend requires only one-fourth the time of galvanic electrolysis alone, making it a popular permanent hair removal technique.

Needle selection

The key to success in permanent hair removal with all types of electrolysis is proper needle insertion. Needles are available in straight, tapered, bulbous, and insulated varieties.[22] Most electrologists prefer to use a straight needle with a gently rounded tip. Tapered needles that are narrower at the tip than the base are sometimes selected for the removal of deep terminal hairs, since more energy can be delivered at the tip without exposing the more superficial tissues to excessive damage.

A variety of needle diameters are also available because the needle diameter must match the diameter of the hair shaft to be treated. Smaller needles generally get hotter than larger needles. Electrologists usually select the largest needle possible to minimize client pain. Needles are generally made of stainless steel in varieties designed for single use or resterilization.

Technique

The technique of the electrologist is important in achieving permanent hair removal without scarring. The most popular technique for needle insertion is known as the forehand technique. The needle holder is held much like a pencil between the thumb and forefinger. The removal forceps are then placed between the needle holder and thumb of the same hand. This allows the free hand to be used for stretching the skin. Skin stretching is important to open the follicular ostia for needle insertion.

The needle is always inserted parallel to the hair shaft opposite to the direction of hair growth. Hairs may exit the skin at angles varying between 10 and 90 degrees. The needle must be inserted at the same angle as hair growth. If the hair is long and lies on the skin surface, it should be clipped to gain a better appreciation of its exit angle. Also, the needle should always be inserted below the hair shaft. These steps are necessary to destroy the follicle without scarring the surrounding skin.

It is important that needle insertion occur to the proper depth. A general rule is that coarse hairs have deeper follicles than fine hairs. A slight dimpling of the overlying skin and resistance means that the bottom of the follicle has been reached and the needle should be withdrawn slightly until the dimpling disappears. A proper needle insertion should be painless and bloodless for the client. Shallow needle insertions may result in pain and scarring for the client.

Once the hair has been treated, the needle should be withdrawn at exactly the same angle as it was inserted. The forceps held between the thumb and needle holder are now positioned 90 degrees to the hair shaft for epilation. The hair should be grasped firmly and should slide gently out of the follicle, if the treatment has been properly performed. Resistance in removing the hair means that the hair has been epilated and not treated with electrolysis, thus regrowth may occur.

Adverse reactions

Electrolysis must be properly performed to minimize patient scarring. Box 9.7 summarizes the pointers that must be followed for successful electrolysis.[23] Care must also be taken to perform the procedure under sanitary conditions to prevent the spread of bacterial and viral infection.[24] The main adverse reaction to electrolysis is pain. The pain can be somewhat minimized by use of the newer topical lidocaine preparations. The technique is not suitable for removal of large hairy areas, such as the male beard. It is most useful in the female with a few unwanted facial hairs on the upper lip or chin, since only 25–100 hairs can be removed per sitting.

REFERENCES

1. Bhaktaviziam C, Mescon H, Matolsky AG. Shaving. *Arch Dermatol* 1963;**88**:242–7.
2. Lynfield YL, MacWilliams P. Shaving and hair growth. J Invest Dermatol 1970;**55**:170–2.
3. Hollander J, Casselman EJ. Factors involved in satisfactory shaving. *JAMA* 1937;**109**:95.

Box 9.7 Electrolysis scar prevention

1. The treated hair should be pulled effortlessly from the follicular ostia.
2. The needle size should be the same as the hair diameter.
3. The skin should be dry.
4. The skin should not blanch following treatment.
5. The current should only flow when the needle has been completely inserted in the follicular ostia to the level of the follicle.
6. The needle should only be removed when the current has stopped.
7. The same follicular ostia should not be reentered or treated twice.

4. Bogaty H. Shaving with razor and blade. Cutis 1978;**21**:609–611.

5. Elden HR. Advances in understanding mechanisms of shaving. *Cosmet Toilet* 1985; **100**: 51–62.

6. Strauss J, Kligman AM. Pseudofolliculitis of the beard. *Arch Dermatol* 1956;**74**:533–42.

7. Spencer TS. Pseudofolliculitis barbae or razor bumps and shaving. *Cosmet Toilet* 1985;**100**:47–9.

8. Brooks GJ, Burmeister F. Preshave and aftershave products. Cosmet Toilet 1990;**105**:67–9.

9. Richards RN, Uy M, Meharg G. Temporary hair removal in patients with hirsuitism: a clinical study. *Cutis* 1990;**45**:199–202.

10. Blackwell G. Ingrown hairs, shaving, and electrolysis. *Cutis* 1977;**19**:172–3.

11. Breuer H. Depilatories. *Cosmet Toilet* 1990; **105**:61–4.

12. de la Guardia M. Facial depilatories on black skin. *Cosmet Toilet* 1976;**91**:37–8.

13. Halder RM. Pseudofolliculitis barbae and related disorders. *Derm Clin* 1988;**6**:407–12.

14. Goldberg HC, Hanfling SL. Hirsutism and electrolysis. *J Med Soc NJ* 1965;**62**:9–14.

15. Richards RN, Meharg GE. *Cosmetic and medical electrolysis and temporary hair removal.* Ontario: Medric Ltd, 1991:17–18.

16. Richards RN, Meharg GE. *Cosmetic and medical electrolysis and temporary hair removal.* Ontario: Medric Ltd, 1991:24–5.

17. Hinkel AR, Lind RW. *Electrolysis, thermolysis and the blend.* California: Arroway Publishers, 1968:181–7.

18. Fino G. *Modern electrology.* New York: Milady Publishing, 1987:35–69.

19. Cipollaro AD. Electrolysis: discussion of equipment, method of operation, indications, contraindications, and warnings concerning its use. *JAMA* 1938;**110**:2488–91.

20. Wagner RF, Tomich JM, Grande DJ. Electrolysis and thermolysis for permanent hair removal. *J Am Acad Dermatol* 1985; **12**:441–9.

21. Hinkel AR, Lind RW. *Electrolysis, thermolysis and the blend.* California: Arroway Publishers, 1968:199–223.

22. Fino G. *Modern electrology.* New York: Milady Publishing, 1987:32–3.

23. Richards RN, Meharg GE. *Cosmetic and medical electrolysis and temporary hair removal.* Ontario: Medric Ltd, 1991:85–6.

24. Petrozzi JW. Verrucae planae spread by electrolysis. *Cutis* 1980;26:85.

10   Tips to maintain healthy hair

Is it possible to increase the longevity of hair? Of course not. Hair is a nonliving tissue that cannot be altered once produced by the follicle. While this is true from a scientific standpoint, it is not true from a cosmetic perspective. Cosmetically, the longevity of hair is determined by how long it remains attached to the head. Thus, anything that causes hair breakage shortens the longevity of the hair shaft. Much industry research is directed at methods of decreasing hair breakage, which is the most common cause of hair loss. In dermatology, we tend to focus on follicular causes of hair loss, such as androgenetic alopecia, female pattern hair loss, alopecia areata, and telogen effluvium, to name some of the most common medically significant causes of hair loss. However, in the hair care industry, issues of grooming friction, cuticle condition, and weathering are evaluated as methods of increasing the longevity of hair.

This chapter deals with methods of increasing the length of time the hair remains attached to the head from a cosmetic perspective by evaluating 10 practical points to share with patients regarding decreased hair breakage. These tips represent a patient-directed summary of some of the main points discussed earlier in this text.

I have called these Zoe's Top 10 Hair Longevity Tips because no extensive studies have been done to document their scientific accuracy and they are based on my own practice experience (Box 10.1). These are the ideas that I share with patients who complain of hair loss on their initial visit to the office, since sometimes I am not ready medically to render a concrete diagnosis until I receive laboratory results or have the patient bring in some lost hair for further analysis. I have found that offering these tips conveys to the patient that I understand hair loss, I am concerned about their problem, and I want to do something immediately to help them while waiting for additional information. Each of these tips is discussed in detail.

Tip 1: Manipulate the hair as little as possible (Figure 10.1)
There is a belief among hairstylists that the more you do to the hair, the healthier it becomes. This is not true. There is no such thing as a 'body restoring permanent wave' or a 'strengthening hair dye.' The more you dye or perm the hair, the weaker it becomes. The more you comb, brush, curl, twist, clip, tease, braid, etc. the hair, the more damage it incurs. This damage is permanent, since the hair is nonliving. Basically, any

Box 10.1 Zoe's Top 10 Hair Longevity Tips

1. Manipulate the hair as little as possible.
2. Select a wide-toothed comb with Teflon-coated tips.
3. Select a vented ball-tipped styling brush.
4. Do not comb wet hair.
5. Allow hair to air-dry avoiding heated drying appliances.
6. Avoid scratching the hair and scalp.
7. Select a conditioning shampoo.
8. Apply an instant conditioner after each shampooing.
9. Consider use of a deep conditioner once weekly.
10. Cut away damaged hair shafts.

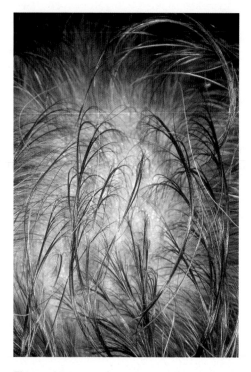

Figure 10.1
Thinning hair that has been manipulated too much will break and appear even thinner.

manipulation of the hair shaft results in the possibility of cuticular damage, which is known in the hair care industry as 'weathering.' Weathering is visible even on the healthiest head of hair as a tightly over-lapped intact cuticle on the newly grown proximal hair shaft, with a disrupted, some-times absent cuticle on the older distal hair shaft. Weathering is basically the sum of chemical and physical environmental insults on the hair shaft, which can be minimized through reduced manipulation.

Tip 2: Select a wide-toothed comb with Teflon-coated tips (Figure 10.2)
One of the most common insults the hair receives on a daily basis is grooming. This grooming is usually done with a comb. Thus, it is important to select a comb that decreases hair breakage by minimizing the friction between the hair and the teeth of the comb. For this reason, a comb should have broadly spaced smooth teeth, preferably Teflon-coated, to reduce combing friction. A comb that tends to grab the hair shafts as they pass through the tangled hair increases hair shaft fracture, usually at the point where cuticular scale is most disrupted or com-pletely absent.

Combing friction is also maximal when the hair shafts are tangled. Unfortunately, the most common reason for combing the hair is to remove tangles. This means that the hair should be protected from situations that might cause hair tangles, such as wind,

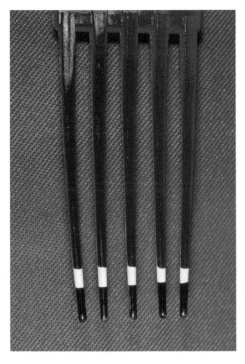

Figure 10.2
A wide-toothed comb should be used to minimize hair shaft breakage, especially when detangling hair after shampooing.

unconscious hair twisting, or teasing. The most effective way to reduce hair combing friction, besides proper comb selection, is application of a conditioner.

Tip 3: Select a vented ball-tipped styling brush (Figure 10.3)

The second most commonly used grooming implement is a brush and it too requires careful selection. The main goal again is to reduce friction between the brush and the hair shafts. Natural bristle brushes or brushes with a dense arrangement of bristles have recently become popular since they fit quite nicely with the current 'back to nature' trend and the use of botanicals in the hair care industry; however, these brushes maximize hair breakage. A better option is to select a brush design, known as a blow-drying brush, for general grooming needs. These brushes possess vents or openings on the brush head to prevent heat from building up between the hair and the brush head. The widely spaced bristles are also plastic and ball-tipped to minimize friction. If drawing the brush across the palm of the hand causes discomfort, the brush is not recommended for use on the hair.

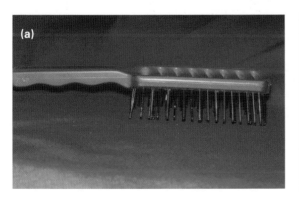
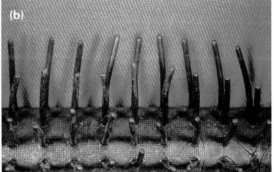

Figure 10.3
(a) A vented ball-tipped blow-drying brush, which minimizes hair breakage from grooming.
(b) A brush without ball tips represents a poor grooming brush choice.

Tip 4: Do not comb wet hair (Figure 10.4)

Hair is much more likely to fracture when wet than when dry. For this reason, it is advisable to gently detangle hair following shampooing from the distal ends to the proximal ends with the fingers, not attempting combing or brushing until the hair is almost dry. Many persons feel that the hair must be styled wet in order to attain the desired style. This is only partially true. Hair will set in the position in which it is placed the instant that the last water molecule evaporates from the hair shaft. This means that the hair is optimally styled just before it is completely dry. Thus, it is best to use fingers to detangle the hair while it is wet and then allow it to almost dry prior to styling to prevent hair breakage.

Tip 5: Allow hair to air-dry avoiding heated drying appliances (Figure 10.5)

Many people prefer to speed the drying process by applying heat to the hair shaft to speed the evaporation of water. This can be done with a hand-held blow-dryer or a hooded professional salon dryer. Heat is

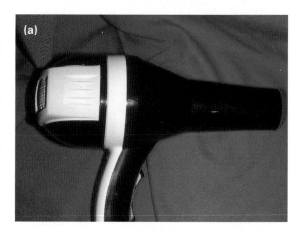

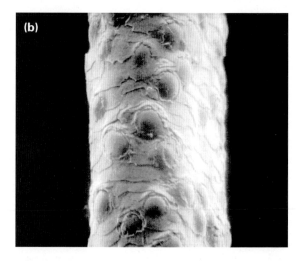

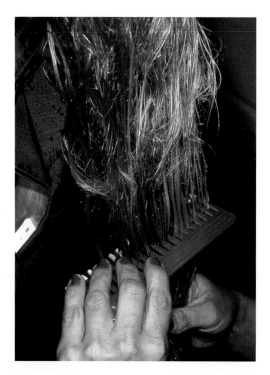

Figure 10.4

Freshly shampooed hair is tangled and fragile, creating a situation conducive to hair shaft fracture.

Figure 10.5

(a) Blow-drying the hair can lead to heat damage and a condition known as bubble hair. (b) An electron micrograph of bubble hair illustrating the bubbles or lumps in the hair shaft caused by escaping steam.

also used to style the hair shafts in the form of heated rollers or a curling iron. Unfortunately, any type of heat that is applied to the hair shafts can permanently damage the protein structure of the hair.

It is important to distinguish between the water that resides on the outside of the hair shaft when the hair is wet and the water that resides inside the hair shaft to act as a plasticizer. Hairdryers attempt to speed evaporation of the water on the outside of the hair shaft and heated styling appliances attempt to rearrange the water deformable bonds within the hair shaft. Remember that water is the plasticizer of all of the keratin-based structures of the body including the skin, hair, and nails. When the hair is rapidly exposed to high temperatures, the water within the shaft turns to steam and exits the hair shaft, creating a loss of cuticular scale and a condition known as 'bubble hair.' Under scanning electron microscopy it is actually possible to see the bubbles created by the energetic steam. Unfortunately, the condition is permanent and bubble hair results in a weakening of the hair shaft that contributes to breakage.

The dermatologist should be aware that many patients who present with hair loss may be experiencing hair breakage due to bubble hair. While it is not possible to see bubble hair under a light microscope, it is possible to have the patient collect 4 days' worth of hair loss, by placing each day's loss in a separate bag. The dermatologist can examine these bags to determine the ratio of broken hairs without the hair bulb to shed telogen hairs containing the hair bulb. If the number of broken hairs exceeds 20%, the patient is experiencing hair breakage. At this point, the dermatologist should inquire as to the use of heated hair-drying and styling appliances and make some recommendations. However, most patients will not discontinue the use of heat.

Even though all forms of heat are damaging to the hair shaft, it is possible to minimize damage by altering the abrupt manner in which the hair comes into contact with heat. Bubble hair is more likely to occur if the room temperature hair shaft is abruptly exposed to high heat. If the hair exposure to the heat is gradual, the damaging effect is not as great. Thus, a gradual temperature increase is recommended. This means that hairdryers can be safely used if the nozzle blowing out hot air is held at least 12 inches from the hair, allowing the air to cool prior to touching the hair shaft. Hairdryers also should be started on low heat to initially warm the hair prior to drying at higher temperatures.

Heated hair rollers and curling irons can be used safely if allowed to cool before application to the hair. These thermostatically controlled devices tend to slightly overheat, which can induce bubble hair immediately on hair contact. Heated styling devices should be unplugged for 1–2 minutes before placing them in contact with the hair. If possible, the styling devices should be operated on a low, rather than high, temperature setting. If the device does not have multiple temperature settings, the temperature of the metal or plastic that contacts the hair can be lowered by placing it in a damp towel. Many patients prefer to use heated styling devices at a high temperature setting, since the high temperature results in the rearrangement of more water deformable bonds and a tighter, longer-lasting curl. Hair that has been heat-damaged appears wavy and friable to the human eye.

Tip 6: Avoid scratching the hair and scalp (Figure 10.6)

It is not usual for patients with seborrheic dermatitis to present with the complaint of hair loss. Medically, it is difficult to reconcile how a fungal infection of the skin of the scalp could alter hair growth from the hair follicles located deep within the dermis and in the superficial subcutaneous tissue. The answer to hair loss in the seborrheic dermatitis patient lies in having the patient collect all hairs lost while shampooing or grooming over a 24-hour period in a bag. Examination of these hairs will reveal absence of the cuticle and hair shaft fracture. Remarkably, it is possible to remove the entire cuticle from the hair shaft with 1 hour of vigorous scratching. Most patients will not scratch their scalp continuously for 1 hour, but the effects of scratching are additive to the hair shaft. One hour can easily be accumulated if the patient scratches 10 minutes a day for 6 days. Usually patients are intending to scratch only the itching present on the scalp, but it is impossible to scratch the scalp without scratching the hair shafts, as well.

Thus, the solution to hair loss in the seborrheic dermatitis patient is to treat the underlying disease. Many times I will treat my patients complaining of hair loss aggressively for scalp puritus in addition to my standard hair loss work-up. Fingernail damage to the hair shaft will result in dull, unmanageable, broken hair that performs poorly. Stopping hair shaft damage from scalp itching is key to solving the cause of hair loss in some patients.

Tip 7: Select a conditioning shampoo (Figure 10.7)

Unfortunately, many patients who present to the dermatologist have already severely damaged their hair and permanent restoration is not possible. Yet, it is important to counsel the patient on how to optimize the

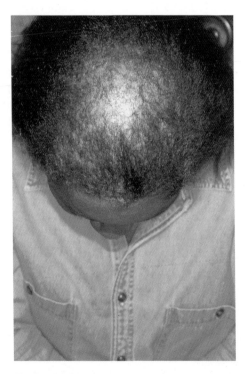

Figure 10.6
Scratching of the scalp can lead to increased hair breakage, magnifying the hair loss characteristic of a scarring alopecia.

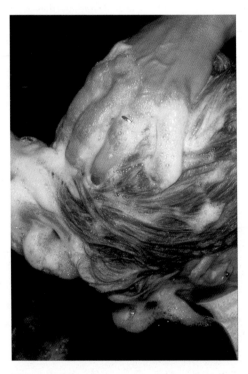

Figure 10.7
Use of a conditioning shampoo can minimize hair shaft damage caused by shampoo detergents.

appearance of their damaged hair until new growth occurs and the damaging cosmetic procedure has been discontinued. One such method of minimizing hair damage is to select a conditioning shampoo. There is no doubt that sebum is the optimal hair conditioner and all synthetic conditioners are a poor substitute; however, patients do not like the greasy, flat appearance sebum imparts to the hair shaft. This led to the introduction of shampoos designed to remove sebum from the hair. Remember that the original intention of shampoo was to remove sebum, skin scale, environmental dirt, and apocrine and eccrine secretions from the scalp. Patients forget that shampoo is to cleanse the scalp and not the hair when they are in the shower.

The need to improve the hair while cleansing the scalp has led to the development of conditioning shampoos. The main ingredient in this technology is silicone, a lightweight clear oil that can coat the hair shaft and smooth the disrupted cuticular scale. This technology was pioneered as part of the Pantene line of shampoos (Procter & Gamble, Cincinnati, OH, USA), still manufactured today. These shampoos were originally known as 2-in-1 shampoos, since they both cleansed the scalp and conditioned the hair. They are available for all types of hair including dry, normal, oily, and chemically treated hair. Silicone is instrumental in these formulas since it can coat the hair shaft without leaving the greasy appearance of sebum. The silicone also significantly reduces the friction of combing and brushing, minimizing hair breakage. Thus, patients with hair loss or chemically damaged hair may benefit from the use of a conditioning silicone-containing shampoo.

Tip 8: Apply an instant conditioner after each shampooing (Figure 10.8)

Silicone technology has also been applied to instant conditioners. Instant conditioners are products applied immediately after shampooing in the bath or shower. They are left on the scalp for a short period of time and then thoroughly rinsed from the hair, hence the name 'instant' conditioner. Since these products do not contain a surfactant designed to remove oils from the scalp, they can focus on augmenting the effect of a previously applied conditioning shampoo. Instant hair conditioners usually incorporate cylomethicone, dimethicone, or amodimethicone as their active agent, in addition to quaternary ammonium compounds. Amodimethicone is a cyclic silicone that appears to have more

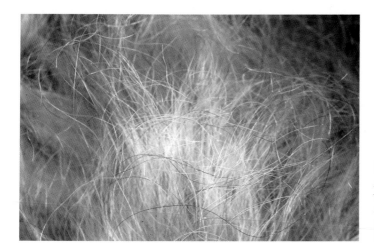

Figure 10.8
An instant conditioner is important to prevent tangles from developing among the hair shafts, which predispose the hair to hair shaft breakage.

substantivity for hair keratin. This means that it sticks to the cuticle better and resists water rinsing, thus providing longer-lasting conditioning. Quaternary ammonium compounds, also known as quats, are excellent at decreasing static electricity, which produces unmanageable frizzy hair.

While these important ingredients function to smooth the loosened cuticular scale and increase hair shine, they also reduce friction. By doing so, it is easier to detangle freshly washed hair, thus reducing hair breakage during the hair-drying process. Hair conditioners also decrease grooming friction between the comb and brush and the hair fibers. Hair conditioners also provide a protective coating over the hair shaft that can protect from heat damage and the effects of UV radiation.

In short, one of the best recommendations the dermatologist can provide to the patient who is experiencing hair loss is to use an instant conditioner following shampooing. Use of this product will prolong hair longevity, no matter what the underlying cause of hair loss may be. No fabrics are sold without a fabric finishing, which improves wear and imparts shine to the fabric. It is actually removal of the fabric finishing that takes a soft cotton T-shirt and changes it into a stiff faded rag with repeated visits to the washing-machine. These same changes occur with hair. Restoring the softness of fabric by using a fabric softener in the washing-machine or dryer is analogous to applying an instant conditioner to the hair.

Tip 9: Consider use of a deep conditioner once weekly (Figure 10.9)

Occasionally it is necessary to impart more conditioning benefits to the hair fiber than an instant conditioner can deliver. This is especially the case in hair that has undergone chemical processing, such as permanent dyeing, bleaching, permanent waving, or chemical straightening. These procedures

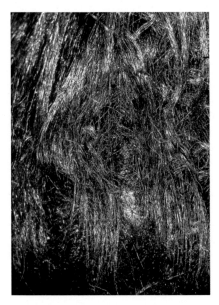

Figure 10.9
Deep conditioners are especially important when chemically straightening African-American hair to prevent hair shaft breakage.

all intentionally disrupt the cuticular scale in order to reach the cortex and medulla of the hair shaft to induce a change in color or configuration. Once the cuticle has been disrupted by chemical processing, it can never be fully restored. Thus, there is a trade-off for the patient between the cosmetic value of chemically treating the hair shaft and its reduced ability to function optimally. Some of the damage can be minimized by using what is known as a deep conditioner.

Deep conditioners are applied to hair for 20–30 minutes outside the bath or shower. They can be used both at home and in a salon. There are basically two types of deep conditioners: oil treatments and protein packs. Oil treatments are usually used for kinky hair that has been straightened. The process of lye straightening hair results in decreased hair water content, which reduces the hair shaft elasticity and predisposes to hair breakage. Applying a heavy oil to the hair shaft is much like moisturizing the skin in that it attempts to both smooth the cuticle and prevent further water loss from the hair shaft. In general, oil treatments are not used for straight hair, since the heavy oil leaves the hair limp and difficult to style.

Protein packs represent a second type of deep conditioner and can be used by all hair types. These conditioners are formulated as creams or lotions and are a variation on the instant conditioner, except that they remain on the hair longer prior to rinsing. Protein packs may contain silicones and quaternary ammonium compounds, as previously discussed, but they also contain some form of hydrolyzed protein. Usually, collagen from animal sources is used, but any hydrolyzed

protein will do. The protein can diffuse into the hair shaft through the cuticular defects created by the chemical treatment. The protein can impart some strength to the hair shaft and also smooth the cuticular scale more thoroughly than an instant conditioner.

For patients who have chemically processed hair, I recommend a deep conditioner once every 1–2 weeks in addition to an instant conditioner after shampooing.

Tip 10: Cut away damaged hair shafts (Figure 10.10)
Many patients who are losing their hair are reluctant to cut their hair. I believe that they feel they should hang onto all their hair in case no more grows. Unfortunately, hair that

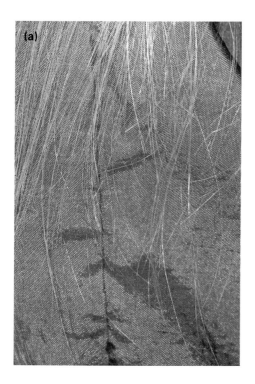
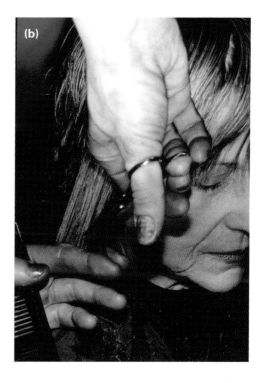

Figure 10.10
(a) Broken irregular hair shafts must be cut away to restore the hair to a presentable appearance, as the hair is nonliving. (b) Patients with thinning hair may be tempted to decrease the frequency of hair trimming. Hair trimming must be performed on an approximately 6-week basis to keep the hair looking full and healthy.

has been damaged by too much chemical processing and too little conditioner application cannot be restored. For these patients, the overall appearance of the hair can be improved simply by removing 1–2 inches from the distal hair shafts. This trims away the split ends and creates new hair ends that are less frizzy, more likely to maintain a curl, and less subject to static electricity. Trimming also eliminates the irregularity of broken hairs that creates a thin appearance. In short, removal of the damaged hair can create the illusion of fuller, healthier hair. Of course, the newly exposed ends must receive proper care or they too will develop an unattractive cosmetic appearance with time.

Summary

Even though hair is a nonliving substance, its 'longevity' can be increased by caring for the hair in an optimal fashion. Much of the product development regarding hair care has been the adaptation of textile processing techniques to the human hair fiber. When hair is thought of as a fabric, it is easy to understand how proper handling of the hair fiber and limited exposure to damaging chemicals and environmental variables can influence its cosmetic performance. This chapter has discussed in an organized fashion the suggestions I give to patients who are experiencing hair loss either totally or partially related to hair breakage.

11 Recommended reading for consumers

Patients frequently request books to read regarding hairstyling ideas and techniques. This text has presented hair care from a medical perspective for the physician. The texts listed here present hair care from a consumer perspective that may be helpful for patients.

Barrick-Hickey B. *500 Beauty solutions*. Naperville, IL: Sourcebooks, 1994.
Barrick-Hickey B. *1001 Beauty solutions*. Napersville, IL: Sourcebooks, 1995.
Campsie J. *Hair & make-up*. British Columbia: Whitecapp Books, 1998.
Painell C, Cameron E. *Cosmopolitan short cuts to looking good*. Toronto: Stoddart Publishing, 1989.
These texts are full of tips as to how to style and care for hair.

Punches L. *How to simply cut hair*. South Lake Tahoe, CA: Punches Productions, 1989.
Bent B. *How to cut your own or anybody else's hair*. New York: Simon and Schuster, 1975.
These texts are an excellent reference for the patient wishing to cut their own hair or the hair of family members.

Coen P, Maxwell J. *Beautiful braids*. New York: Prince Paperbacks Crown Publishers, 1984.
The various techniques for braiding hair are presented here in a step-by-step pictorial fashion.

Walk A. *Andre talks hair*. New York: Simon and Schuster, 1997.
Eber J. *Jose Eber beyond hair: the ultimate makeover book*. New York: Simon and Schuster, 1990.
These books written by famous hair stylists present basic hair care ideas for the fashion-conscious patient.

Nardi V, Nardi F. *Color your hair like a pro*. New York: The Putnam Publishing Group, 1986.
Licari L, Esche S. *Color your life . . . with haircolor*. New York: G.P. Putnam's Sons, 1985.
Quant M. *Color be quant*. McGraw-Hill Book Company, 1984.
Hair color selection and dyeing techniques are discussed in these consumer texts.

Mayhew J. *Hair techniques & alternatives to baldness*. New York: Trado-Medic Books, 1983.
This book presents ideas for the patient with thinning hair.

12   Summary

This text has pictorially demonstrated the extensive scientific fund of knowledge regarding hair. The ability to unlock the chemistry of the hair fiber through information borrowed from the textile industry has led to the development of techniques to permanently dye and curl the hair shaft. The creativity of the salon stylist has led to novel ways to cut, comb, and brush the hair into fashion statements of the moment. The ingenuity of the cosmetic chemist has provided new polymers and hair fixatives that can defy gravity and create a multitude of hairstyles for straight, wavy, curly, and kinky hair. All of these techniques provide additional outlets for personal expression through the appearance of scalp hair.

It is interesting to note that humans are the only higher level mammalian society where scalp hair is considered desirable. In the power hierarchy of the adult ape, the most senior ape is identified by the fact that his pate is bald! His lack of scalp hair indicates that he is the oldest ape and his life experiences are used by the rest of the younger apes to guide the group through the dangerous forest safely. Sociologic experiments have been done where a toupee is placed on the bald eldest ape and the clan no longer follows his lead. Somehow, in our society, we value the youthful appearance of scalp hair more than the wisdom that accompanies baldness. This has led to the development of medications to prevent baldness, hair addition techniques, and a variety of wigs. These methods of treating baldness also become a part of the cosmetic arena surrounding hair.

It is hoped that this text has left visual impressions supplemented by words to enable the physician to better understand the many issues surrounding scalp hair. Hair is indeed a fascinating material used to establish gender, age, and personal style. Our hair says a great deal about how we perceive ourselves and how we wish to be perceived by those around us. Hair is indeed a fascinating study into the values and ideals of a society. This atlas has examined the scientific aspects of the keratin structure affectionately known as hair.

13　Index

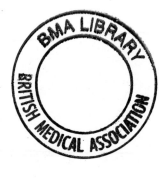